Medical Emergency Training Simulations for Dental Teams:

Four Years of Monthly First Aid Simulations for Unshakeable Confidence and Professional Excellence

T.M. Donnelly

ISBN: 978-1-0695998-0-3

This book includes access to additional online content, featuring printable assessment forms and training records.
Register your book or book at
www.learn-online.northcoast.academy/book-resources
and follow the prompts to get access

This book is intended for educational and training purposes only. Every effort has been made to ensure that the information presented is accurate, current, and based on reputable sources and professional guidelines available at the time of publication. However, medical knowledge and practice continually evolve, and it remains the responsibility of the reader to use sound clinical judgment and consult current standards of care, regulatory requirements, and professional guidelines when applying any of the information contained herein. The author and publisher expressly disclaim any liability for loss, injury, or damage incurred, directly or indirectly, as a result of the use or misuse of the information contained in this publication. The simulations and scenarios are illustrative and educational tools—not a substitute for proper training, clinical experience, or professional medical advice. By using this material, the reader acknowledges and agrees to these terms.

For my family.

Introduction to Simulation Training

Simulations

Get Started!

Prologue

In the dynamic environment of a modern dental practice, excellence is defined not only by clinical expertise but by preparedness for the unexpected.

Monthly medical emergency training represents far more than a regulatory checkbox—it embodies your commitment to the highest standard of patient care. When a medical crisis unfolds in your operatory, the difference between a controlled response and chaos lies in the muscle memory developed through consistent, deliberate practice. By implementing monthly emergency drills, your team transforms theoretical knowledge into intuitive action, creating a seamless response system that protects patients and elevates your practice above the competition.

The ripple effects of regular emergency preparedness extend throughout your entire practice ecosystem. Patients sense and value the confidence that radiates from a well-trained team, building the trust that drives referrals and practice growth. Staff members experience heightened professional satisfaction knowing they possess life-saving capabilities that transcend routine dental procedures. Insurance carriers recognize and reward practices demonstrating proactive risk management. Perhaps most significantly, regular emergency training fosters an environment where team members communicate effectively, support one another under pressure, and share a profound commitment to excellence. This collective competence becomes your practice's signature—a reputation for exceptional care that distinguishes you in an increasingly competitive marketplace. By embracing monthly emergency preparedness, you're not just preparing for rare events; you're cultivating the clinical confidence, team cohesion, and professional distinction that define truly outstanding dental practices.

Introduction to Simulation Training

- Assessing Team Performance - Feedback and Debriefing with STAT-DO
- Practice Frequency and Records
- Creating High-Fidelity Simulations
- Training Supplies for Emergency Simulations

Assessing Team Performance - Feedback and Debriefing with STAT-DO

Simulation-based training is a cornerstone of preparing dental teams for the rare but critical medical emergencies that can occur in a dental practice. While high-fidelity simulations offer experiential learning, their full educational value depends on the provision of effective feedback and structured assessment. To this end, the use of standardized, valid, and reliable assessment tools is essential.

Why Assessment Matters in Simulation-Based Education

In the context of medical simulation, assessment is not merely a scorecard—it is an educational tool. It provides structure for debriefing, guides learner reflection, and anchors instructor feedback in observable behaviours. Without structured assessment, feedback can become subjective, inconsistent, or overly general, which limits learning.

From an educational theory perspective, Miller's Pyramid of Clinical Competence offers a useful framework. It describes four levels of clinical learning:

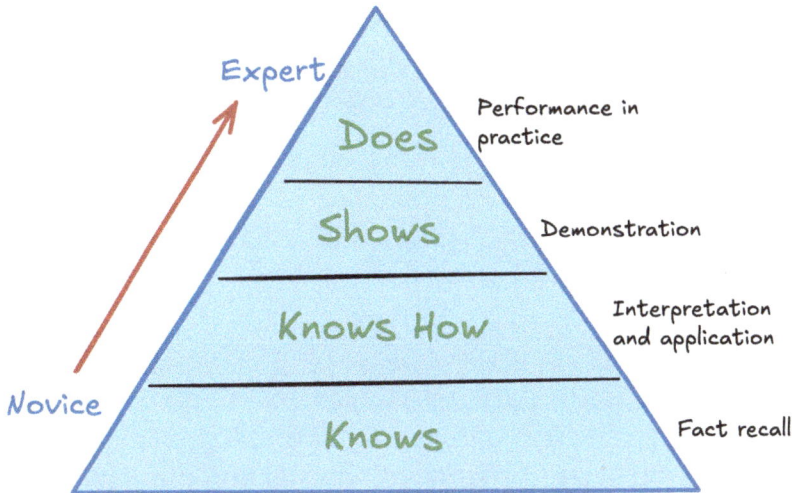

- Knows (basic knowledge),

- Knows how (applied knowledge),

- Shows how (performance in simulated environments),

- Does (actual clinical performance).

Simulation occupies the critical "shows" or "shows how" level, where learners demonstrate application of knowledge and skills in a controlled but realistic context. Structured assessment tools like STAT-DO allow instructors to evaluate performance at this level, providing meaningful insights into a learner's readiness for real-world emergencies.

Furthermore, assessment instruments promote constructive alignment, ensuring that the learning objectives, instructional methods, and evaluation strategies all reinforce one another. If the goal is to improve interprofessional emergency response in the dental office, then the assessment must focus on team dynamics, communication, leadership, and situational awareness— not just individual procedural skills.

Origin and Purpose of the STAT Tool

The original Simulation Team Assessment Tool (STAT)[1] was developed to evaluate team performance during medical simulation scenarios in hospital and prehospital settings. It was designed with ease of use in mind, allowing instructors to assess teams across core non-technical skills: leadership, communication, situational awareness, resource utilization, and clinical judgment. The tool utilizes a 2-point Likert scale for each domain, providing space for narrative comments that promote both quantitative scoring and qualitative feedback.

Importantly, STAT was designed for real-time or post-event assessment by simulation facilitators. It has been used in various healthcare education contexts, including emergency medicine, anaesthesia, and critical care, and it aligns closely with Crisis Resource Management (CRM) principles—skills that are directly transferable to dental office emergencies.

Why STAT-DO? Rationale for Adaptation to Dental Simulation

While dental emergencies are infrequent, their management demands rapid, coordinated action under pressure. Dental teams are often small, and the roles are less rigidly defined than in hospitals, making team communication and role clarity even more critical. An assessment tool for this setting must reflect the realities of the dental environment while retaining the rigour of a validated evaluation framework.

The STAT-DO (Dental Office) version of the tool has been adapted to reflect:

- The typical structure and scope of dental teams,

- Common medical emergencies encountered in dentistry (e.g. vasovagal syncope, anaphylaxis, hypoglycemia, cardiac arrest),

- The emphasis on shared responsibility since leadership in dental offices is often collaborative,

- The need for prompt activation of external EMS resources.

Each domain in STAT-DO focuses on observable behaviours during simulation, which supports both formative feedback during debriefing and summative assessment for tracking improvement over time. The tool's simplicity allows for consistent use by a variety of educators, including those without formal training in assessment theory.

Including a tool like STAT-DO in your simulation training program moves your educational efforts from ad hoc practice to structured, evidence-informed education. It reinforces the key competencies that teams must demonstrate during medical emergencies and supports learners in developing the non-technical skills essential for safe and effective care.

In the high-stakes moments of a true dental emergency, it's not just about who knows what to do—it's about whether the team can work together effectively under pressure. STAT-DO helps ensure that your training prepares them to do exactly that.

Validity, Reliability, and Practical Utility

In educational measurement, validity refers to whether an instrument truly measures what it claims to measure, and reliability refers to the consistency of that measurement across different raters and scenarios. The original STAT tool has shown good inter-rater reliability and content validity in healthcare simulation literature. While the STAT-DO version requires further formal study, its design principles follow the same framework.

By providing a consistent structure, STAT-DO enables:

- Objective comparison across simulation sessions,

- Targeted feedback aligned with performance gaps,

- Data collection for quality improvement or credentialing,

- Self-assessment and reflective practice for learners.

How to Use the STAT-DO Tool

The STAT-DO tool is designed to be both simple and structured, allowing simulation facilitators to assess team performance during dental office emergency scenarios in real time or immediately afterward. Its purpose is not to "pass or fail" learners but to support feedback, reflection, and ongoing improvement in how dental teams respond to crisis situations.

As with the original STAT Tool, the scoring for the STAT-DO is behaviourally anchored. Two points are awarded if the skill is completed and timely, one point is awarded if the skill is performed but incomplete or untimely, and zero points are awarded if the skill needs to be performed, but was not performed or was performed incorrectly. This relatively simple scoring scheme helps preserve the reliability of the scale.

An example of scoring on the scale can be drawn from a patient who requires an IV to be established and fluid to be administered. In this case, the learner would score 2 points for completing the IV correctly and administering fluid. They would receive only one point if they established the IV, but it took them several attempts to do so or if they established the IV but forgot to administer the fluid. Finally, the learner would receive zero points if they failed to recognize the need for the IV and did not start it, or if they attempted to start it but were completely unsuccessful.

Timing and Context

The STAT-DO tool can be used during a live simulation or retrospectively after observing video recordings. It is best used during high-fidelity or moderately realistic scenarios that simulate medical emergencies such as anaphylaxis, cardiac arrest, hypoglycemia, or airway compromise. Facilitators should familiarize themselves with the specific roles and layout of the dental office involved to better interpret team actions.

Observer Role

One designated instructor or evaluator should act as the primary observer, completing the tool without presenting the simulation or intervening during the simulation. The observer uses the six performance domains to guide their attention: leadership, communication, coordination, situational awareness, clinical problem-solving, and overall performance. Each domain includes example behaviours to clarify what constitutes poor, acceptable, or excellent performance.

Observers should aim to assign a numerical score (0,1, or 2) for each domain and jot down specific behavioural examples under the comments section. This will support focused feedback during debriefing.

Debriefing Integration

Following the simulation, STAT-DO becomes a debriefing scaffold. The facilitator can use the domains as talking points:

"Let's talk about how roles were assigned and how leadership was communicated…"

"What did you notice about your situational awareness when the patient's condition changed?"

This approach allows the debrief to move beyond factual errors and toward critical non-technical skills that affect real-world outcomes.

Fidelity and Timing

It can be useful to record a note about the level of fidelity for each simulation as it was performed (high, medium, low) to help contextualize performance scores. For example, a team struggling in a low-fidelity environment may still demonstrate strong reasoning or communication that deserves recognition.

The section titled "Time to Key Interventions" allows instructors to track how quickly life-saving actions (e.g. administration of epinephrine, CPR initiation) were performed. This can be useful for both benchmarking performance and identifying delays due to hesitation, confusion, or unclear roles.

Flexibility and Adaptability

STAT-DO can be used with interprofessional teams, including dentists, assistants, hygienists, and office staff. While it's tailored for team assessment, it can also support individual performance review by noting specific contributions or areas for growth. Over time, repeated use of the tool across different scenarios can help identify patterns in team dynamics or persistent learning needs.

By incorporating STAT-DO into your simulation sessions, you ensure that your evaluation of performance is consistent, educationally grounded, and directly tied to the skills that matter most in real emergencies: teamwork, clarity, and rapid decision-making.

Simulation Team Assessment Tool for the Dental Office (STAT-DO)

Adapted from the Simulation Team Assessment Tool (STAT)

Scenario Title:	
Facilitator Name:	
Date:	
Rating Scale	
1 = Poor – Ineffective or absent	
2 = Marginal – Needs improvement	
3 = Acceptable – Meets expectations	
4 = Good – Some strengths evident	
5 = Excellent – Highly effective	

1. Leadership & Role Assignment

Was a clear leader identified?

Did the leader guide the team calmly and effectively?

Were roles (e.g., airway management, medication prep, calling 911) clearly delegated?

Score (1-5):

1	2	3	4	5

Comments

2. Communication
Was communication clear, concise, and timely?
Did the team use closed-loop communication?
Were critical decisions verbalized for team awareness?

Score (1-5):

1	2	3	4	5

Comments

3. Team Coordination & Resource Utilization
Did team members anticipate needs and assist one another?
Were available resources (e.g., AED, emergency kit, EMS activation) used appropriately?
Did the team avoid duplication of tasks?

Score (1-5):

1	2	3	4	5

Comments

4. Situational Awareness
Did the team monitor the patient's condition and environment effectively?
Were changes in patient status recognized and acted upon?
Was there awareness of time-sensitive actions (e.g., oxygen, epinephrine, CPR)?

Score (1-5):

1	2	3	4	5

Comments

5. Clinical Problem Solving
Was the underlying medical emergency correctly identified?
Were treatments appropriate and timely (e.g., glucose for hypoglycemia, epinephrine for anaphylaxis)?
Did the team adjust their approach as the scenario evolved?

Score (1-5):

1	2	3	4	5

Comments

6. Overall Team Performance
Did the team function cohesively under pressure?
Was patient care safe and appropriate?
Would you feel confident in this team's ability to manage a real emergency?

Score (1-5):

1	2	3	4	5

Comments

Facilitator Reflection Notes
Strengths observed:

Areas for improvement:

Debrief focus points:

Time to key interventions:

Time	Intervention

To download a printable copy, use the instructions at the front of this book to access the online resources.

Practice Frequency and Records

Regular monthly practice in managing medical emergencies is essential for every dental office committed to patient safety and professional excellence.

Consistent training ensures your team responds quickly and confidently when seconds count, transforming preparedness into a competitive advantage that builds trust and strengthens your practice's reputation.

To support this ongoing commitment, this chapter includes checklists designed to document each training session. These checklists serve as a clear record of your team's progress, helping you maintain accountability, meet regulatory requirements, and continuously improve your emergency response skills.

Together, regular practice and thorough documentation empower your dental office to stand out as a leader in patient care and safety.

Medical Emergency Training Record

Simulation/Scenario Name:
Date of Training:
Participants (Names & Roles):
1.
2.
3.
4.
5.
6.
7.
8.
Equipment or Infrastructure Needs Identified: (List any supplies, equipment, or facility issues discovered during the simulation)
Trainer/Facilitator Signature:

To download a printable copy, use the instructions at the front of this book to access the online resources.

Creating High-Fidelity Simulations

High-fidelity simulation is widely recognized as a powerful tool in healthcare education. In the context of dental office emergencies, high-fidelity scenarios enable dental professionals to rehearse the recognition and management of life-threatening events in an environment that closely resembles their actual clinical practice. But what exactly is fidelity, and how do we achieve "high fidelity" in a busy dental office with limited time and resources?

What is Fidelity?

In simulation-based education, fidelity refers to the degree to which a simulation replicates the real world. This includes not only the visual realism (e.g. a lifelike mannequin) but also psychological and contextual realism —how real the scenario feels to participants in terms of decision-making, pressure, and engagement.

There are three major dimensions of fidelity:

- Physical fidelity: The extent to which the simulation looks and feels like a real clinical environment (e.g.

equipment, mannequins, patient monitors).

- Psychological fidelity: The degree to which participants are emotionally and cognitively engaged—feeling like it "really matters"

- Procedural (or "Functional") fidelity: How accurately the scenario mimics real-world task demands and workflow, such as calling 911, delegating roles, or administering emergency medications.

High-fidelity simulations don't require expensive equipment. Instead, they need thoughtful design, contextual realism, and clear learning objectives.

Why Fidelity Matters

The more realistic a simulation feels, the more likely learners are to behave as they would in a real emergency. This enhances:

- Transfer of learning: Skills practiced in simulation are more likely to be recalled and applied correctly in actual events.

- Engagement and buy-in: Learners take the training seriously when it feels authentic.

- Assessment accuracy: Realistic scenarios reveal true team dynamics, knowledge gaps, and decision-making under pressure.

From a theoretical standpoint, Kolb's experiential learning theory suggests that learners progress through a cycle of experience, reflection, conceptualization, and experimentation.[2] Fidelity enhances the experiential component, providing a foundation for deep reflection and behaviour change.

Practical Approaches for Dental Office Simulations

Not every simulation session requires a high-tech mannequin or an elaborate setup. In fact, many dental offices conduct in-situ training (simulation in the actual workspace) to promote realistic practice using everyday tools and familiar team configurations. Here are some strategies to maximize fidelity within realistic constraints:

1. Use the Actual Clinical Environment

Conduct simulations in a real operatory using the office's own emergency equipment.

Involve actual staff members in their usual roles.

Maintain the usual layout and workflow, including the use of intercoms or phones to call EMS.

2. Create Realistic Scenarios, Not Just Realistic Props

Focus on common emergencies like syncope, anaphylaxis, angina, hypoglycemia, or cardiac arrest.

Use a well-written case stem that encourages learners to gather cues, assess the information, and make a decision, rather than simply following a checklist.

Allow the scenario to evolve based on participant actions,

simulating real-life unpredictability.

3. Use Simple Props Thoughtfully

A basic CPR mannequin with a removable oxygen mask can represent a patient.

Use moulage sparingly—for example, some simple red Hallowe'en makeup to indicate a rash for anaphylaxis or a sticker to simulate an insulin pump.

Consider using voice-of-the-patient techniques (a facilitator voicing symptoms from behind a barrier or screen).

4. Rehearse with Role-Players

Have a facilitator or actor role-play a distressed family member or patient to add emotional realism.

Alternatively, use a "silent patient" mannequin but simulate breathing, pulse, and responsiveness through prompts or monitors.

5. Leverage Low-Tech Audio-Visual Cues

Play pre-recorded sounds (e.g. gasping, coughing, alarms).

Display a patient monitor graphic on a tablet or laminated card.

Use phone props or radios to simulate making a call to EMS.

6. Keep the Time Commitment Realistic

A high-fidelity simulation can be run in 15–20 minutes, followed by a focused debrief.

Focus on one or two learning objectives per session (e.g. recognition of cardiac arrest, role clarity in emergencies).

Use "micro-simulations" if needed—brief scenarios embedded in morning huddles or lunch-and-learns.

Fidelity is a Design Decision

Ultimately, fidelity is not an all-or-nothing proposition. It is a strategic choice, tailored to the goals of the session, the resources available, and the culture of the dental team. You can create high psychological and functional fidelity even with modest physical resources.

Remember, the most effective simulations feel urgent, relevant, and emotionally resonant. A simple scenario, executed thoughtfully, can have more educational impact than an elaborate production with no emotional engagement.

Training Supplies for Emergency Simulation

B y the end of this chapter, readers will be able to:

- Identify essential and optional training supplies for conducting in-office medical emergency simulations.
- Understand how to select and maintain cost-effective, safe, and feasible simulation props.
- Strike a balance between fidelity and simplicity to promote regular training.
- Build a simulation kit that supports monthly team-based drills without becoming burdensome.

Introduction

Purpose of Simulation Supplies

The use of simulation in dental offices is a powerful tool for preparing teams to respond effectively to medical emergencies. While the scenarios themselves provide structure and learning objectives, it's the simulation supplies, the props, moulage, and mock medications, that can help bring the experience to life!
Used well, these items enhance realism, deepen immersion, and help participants suspend disbelief just enough to behave as they would in a real emergency.

When participants can physically interact with training tools —such as administering a mock dose of epinephrine, applying a mask, or reading 'vital signs' from a monitor card—they are more likely to retain procedural steps, refine teamwork behaviors, and internalize their roles during an actual crisis.

Having a dedicated, ready-to-use set of training supplies increases the educational value of simulation and reduces cognitive load during training. It signals to the team that simulation is a regular, professional exercise—part of the office's safety culture, not an occasional novelty.

A Philosophy of Simplicity and Feasibility

A common barrier to conducting simulations regularly is the misconception that realism must come at the cost of complexity and expense. This chapter embraces a different approach: "good enough to train effectively." You do not need hospital-grade mannequins or high-end moulage kits to run valuable simulations. You need props that are recognizable, safe, and functional, and a setup that is practical within the time, space, and budget constraints of a dental office.

Simplicity in simulation design allows for greater consistency in training. A plastic pill bottle labelled "nitroglycerine" may not be photorealistic, but if it reinforces proper medication delivery in a time-critical situation, it's doing its job. Using a CPR mannequin to simulate a patient with asthma or seizure is also perfectly acceptable when paired with realistic scenario cues and role play. The goal is not to impress with special effects, but to foster decision-making, communication, and readiness through hands-on repetition.

Encouraging Routine Practice

For simulations to have a lasting impact, they must happen regularly. Monthly training sessions, even as brief as 15–30 minutes in length, can significantly enhance a team's ability to respond to emergencies. However, if setting up a simulation feels like a burden, requiring extensive prep time or delicate equipment, it will become one more thing pushed to the bottom of the to-do list.

The training supplies discussed in this chapter are selected and recommended with routine, low-barrier use in mind. They are designed to be stored in a single bin, drawer, or tote that can be easily pulled out and used with minimal setup. These tools should reduce friction, not create it. When your supplies are simple, safe, affordable, and reusable, they become an enabler, not an obstacle, to building a confident, competent team that is ready to act when it matters most.

Core Principles for Selecting Training Supplies

Before investing in simulation supplies for your dental office, it's essential to understand the guiding principles that will help you choose items that are safe, effective, and sustainable. These principles are designed to support training that is practical, impactful, and repeatable.

Safety First

Safety must be the foundational principle when selecting any training material. While simulation is a low-risk educational activity, inappropriate supplies can still pose hazards or cause confusion in a clinical environment.

- *Avoid Sharps and Real Medications*: Never include needles, expired medications, or working medical devices in your training kit. Even if "out of date," these items could pose a risk if misused or mistaken for active stock.

- *Use Clearly Labelled Training Items*: All simulation supplies should be marked as "TRAINING ONLY". This includes mock medications, oxygen masks, and any repurposed medical devices. Labelling helps prevent clinical staff from accidentally using training materials in patient care, particularly during emergencies. Despite our best intentions, distractions occur, and some of these materials may end up left out on a counter somewhere, potentially causing hazardous confusion.

- *Prevent Cross-Contamination*: Avoid reusing items like mannequin face pieces or simulation airway devices between team members without proper cleaning. Infection control best practices should be followed.

By prioritizing safety, you maintain trust in the simulation process and prevent unintended consequences from well-meaning but misapplied training efforts.

Fidelity vs. Functionality

In simulation, fidelity refers to the degree to which a simulation accurately represents the real world. It can be broken into a few categories. We talked about this earlier but here is a quick recap:

- *Physical fidelity*: How realistic the props or mannequins appear (e.g. lifelike facial expressions, accurate anatomy).

- *Emotional fidelity*: How much the simulation engages the participants emotionally and psychologically.

- *Procedural (Functional) fidelity*: How closely the tasks mimic the steps required in a real emergency.

While high-fidelity mannequins and props can be impressive, they are often expensive and unnecessary for office-based simulation. In a dental setting, functionality is far more important than photorealism.
For example:

- A labelled plastic pill bottle can effectively simulate nitroglycerine delivery.

- A paper monitor with printed vital signs can prompt appropriate clinical responses.

- A team member describing symptoms out loud can be more powerful than any moulage makeup.

Use high fidelity selectively, when it adds educational value, such as using makeup for a swollen airway or creating a realistic tremor effect during a seizure drill. For everything else, prioritize clarity and utility. Keep your focus on behaviour, communication, and decision-making over visual perfection.

Cost and Accessibility

One of the key advantages of in-office simulation is that it can be done affordably and accessibly. You do not need a large budget to make training effective.

- *Use what you already have*: CPR mannequins, expired (non-hazardous) supplies, printed materials, or classroom props can all be repurposed.

- *Creative substitutions*: Empty medication vials, colour-coded labels, and laminated vitals cards can all simulate essential components of emergency care without requiring advanced technology.

- *Digital aids*: Free or inexpensive apps can simulate monitor beeping, oxygen saturation tones, or patient audio cues to add realism without incurring additional costs.

Use an incremental approach to building your simulation kit: Start with a few essential items (e.g. mock medications, a mannequin, printed vital signs). Gradually add functional upgrades (e.g. moulage kit, printed labels, scenario cards), and reevaluate regularly and replace or add items as needed. This approach keeps your kit small, uncluttered, minimally expensive and maximally useful.

Ease of Storage, Setup, and Reset

The biggest threat to consistent simulation is logistical hassle. If it takes too long to gather, set up, and put away training materials, the simulation will fall by the wayside.

Your supplies should be:

- *Compact and portable*: A single labelled tote, bin, or drawer should hold most or all items.

- *Pre-organized*: Keep props grouped into small kits by scenario (e.g. "chest pain," "seizure,""airway emergency") so staff can grab what they need without digging.

- *Quick to deploy and repack*: Aim for a setup and teardown time of under 10 minutes to make monthly simulation practical.

Designating a simulation coordinator or, at the very least, assigning the kit maintenance role to someone in the office can help keep supplies organized and readily available. This way, conducting a drill becomes a quick and manageable task, rather than an overwhelming project.

Essential Simulation Kit Contents

A well-equipped, yet manageable simulation kit can dramatically increase the efficiency and effectiveness of your monthly training sessions.

The following sections outline the core items every dental office should consider including. These supplies are selected for their utility, affordability, and ease of use in realistic, office-based scenarios. Most items can be repurposed from existing training materials or sourced at minimal cost.

This kit is designed to be compact enough to store in a

single tote or drawer and quick enough to set up in under 10 minutes.

Basic Props (Essential for Monthly Drills)

These core items provide the foundational tools necessary to run realistic medical emergency simulations. They enable hands-on practice of critical steps, reinforce muscle memory, and simulate the physical components of patient care.

Airway Trainer or Basic CPR Torso: It is not always comfortable or appropriate to use a staff member to act as the sick person. A standard CPR mannequin is often sufficient for most simulations, especially those involving airway emergencies, cardiac arrest, or unconscious patients. If available, a basic airway trainer enables more advanced demonstrations, such as airway positioning or suction simulation.

Mock Medications: Use empty, clearly labelled vials and containers to simulate emergency medications such as:

- Epinephrine (auto-injectors or ampoules)
- Nitroglycerine (spray or tablet bottle)
- Oral glucose gel or tubes
- Glucagon kits (mock or expired trainers).

These should be distinctly marked "TRAINING ONLY" and stored away from active clinical stock.

- *Oxygen Delivery Supplies*: Nasal cannulas, simple oxygen masks, and bag-valve-mask devices (BVMs) can add realism to airway and respiratory emergency scenarios. These are often available as expired or demo units from medical suppliers.

- *Vital Sign Indicators*: Use printed monitor "snapshots" with vital signs corresponding to the scenario (e.g. tachycardia in anaphylaxis, bradycardia in overdose). Alternatively, simple apps or audio recordings can simulate the sounds of pulse oximeter beeps, cardiac alarms, or agonal breathing. Whatever you decide to use, it should reflect the information and equipment that will be available in your dental clinic during a real emergency. (Don't introduce 12-lead ECGs into a scenario if your clinic doesn't even have a cardiac monitor.)

- *Paper Charts / Scenario Cards:* Include basic paper materials that assign roles (e.g. team leader, recorder, airway manager) or provide scenario background (e.g. "patient collapsed while in chair," "complains of chest pressure"). These tools guide participants and provide structure without requiring technology.

Simple Moulage Supplies

Moulage refers to the use of makeup or visual cues to simulate injuries, illnesses, or physical symptoms. While not essential for every drill, simple moulage can enhance immersion and help participants recognize visual clues during assessment.

Fake Blood and Makeup Kits: Use theatrical makeup or Halloween-grade kits to simulate bruising, cyanosis, flushed skin, or bleeding. Modelling clay in skin tones can mimic swelling (e.g. facial edema in anaphylaxis).

Symptom Cards and Labels: Place index cards or sticky labels on the "patient" (a mannequin or actor) to simulate symptoms that aren't easily visualized. Examples:

- "Patient is sweating profusely"
- "Slurred speech"
- "One pupil is dilated"

These cards prompt responders to ask questions and interpret the cues as part of their assessment.

Patient Actor Accessories: Simple props, such as wigs, reading glasses, or scarves, can help represent different patients and avoid a sense of repetition. These are particularly helpful when rotating staff into patient roles.

Facilitator Tools

To guide, observe, and evaluate the simulation effectively, the facilitator needs a few key tools. These materials help track time, prompt learning objectives, and support structured debriefing.

Timer or Stopwatch: Used to time the scenario or track response intervals (e.g. "Time to first epinephrine administration"). This is useful for benchmarking improvement over time.

Clipboards and Debrief Notes: Facilitators can jot down observations during the scenario, noting both strengths and areas for improvement. This also encourages professional reflection and supports learning conversations during the debrief.

Laminated Evaluation Forms or Dry-Erase Boards:
Evaluation forms can be customized to your office protocols and reused for each drill. Dry-erase boards are helpful for quickly jotting down scenario notes or simulating documentation in real-time.

By assembling these basic components, your dental office will be well-equipped to conduct engaging, high-impact simulations without the need for expensive equipment or complex logistics. Later in this chapter, we'll explore optional upgrades that can further enhance your training, if and when your team is ready to expand.

Overcoming Common Barriers

Despite the best intentions, many dental offices struggle to maintain consistent simulation training over time. The most common obstacles are not a lack of interest or importance, but logistical and psychological barriers that can make simulation feel inconvenient, intimidating, or unnecessary.

This section offers practical, low-friction solutions to help your team overcome these challenges and stay committed to a sustainable training routine.

Barrier: "The supplies are too expensive."

Solution: Embrace low-cost or DIY alternatives.

Simulation does not require expensive equipment to be effective. You can achieve high-quality training outcomes with:

- Printed vital sign charts instead of electronic

monitors
- Empty, labelled vials in place of real medications
- Reused CPR mannequins instead of high-fidelity simulators
- Household items (makeup, modelling clay) for moulage effects

Start small with core items, then upgrade only as your budget and engagement grow. Consider sharing resources with nearby dental offices or training partners, or reaching out to your local dental society for support.

Barrier: "Setting up is too time-consuming."

Solution: Pre-organize and simplify the setup.

Time constraints are one of the most common reasons simulation gets skipped. However, with a well-organized kit, setup and teardown can be completed in under 10 minutes.
Tips:

- Pre-sort scenario kits into labelled bags (e.g. "Seizure Drill," "Chest Pain Drill")
- Store all supplies in one clearly labelled container
- Keep printed facilitator guides and scenario prompts with the kit

Assigning a Simulation Coordinator can also streamline the process and take pressure off clinical staff.

Barrier: "We mixed up training items with real supplies."

Solution: Use clear, prominent labelling.

Avoiding cross-contamination between simulation and clinical supplies is critical for safety and clarity.
All training items—especially anything resembling medication or oxygen delivery—should be labelled:

"TRAINING ONLY, NOT FOR CLINICAL USE"

Consider using coloured tape or laminated tags. Storing the simulation kit in a dedicated, separate location also helps prevent mix-ups.

Barrier: "It's not realistic enough to be valuable."

Solution: Use verbal cues, props, and scenario framing to enhance immersion.

While visual realism helps, the most powerful realism comes from engagement. Use these techniques to enhance the training experience:

- Provide symptom cards (e.g. "patient is slurring words," "breathing rapidly")
- Use roleplay: Have a team member act as the patient, complete with accessories or voice changes
- Play ambient sounds (e.g. monitor tones, wheezing) using a smartphone and Bluetooth speaker

Remember: It's not about movie-quality effects—it's about giving the team a believable context to rehearse life-saving behaviours.

Barrier: "Nobody has time to run simulations."

Solution: Keep it brief and schedule it.

Effective simulations don't need to be long. A well-run drill can be:

- 10–15 minutes for the scenario
- 10–15 minutes for the debrief

In under 30 minutes, your team can review critical protocols, practice communication, and reflect on their performance.

Make it easy by:

- Scheduling simulations on slow days or lunch hours
- Combining them with monthly staff meetings
- Rotating facilitator roles to share the workload

Consistency is more important than complexity. Regular short drills are better than infrequent, elaborate ones.

Overcoming these barriers means shifting the mindset from perfection to practicality. Simulation does not require Hollywood-level performances—it's about building confidence, readiness, and muscle memory in the setting where emergencies are most likely to occur: your own dental office.

Maintenance and Storage Tips

A well-designed simulation kit can serve your team for years if it is properly maintained, stored, and routinely refreshed. Just like clinical tools, your training supplies require organization, oversight, and occasional replacement to remain safe, functional, and ready for use. This section offers practical strategies to ensure your kit remains reliable and your simulations run smoothly.

Designate a Storage Space

One of the most significant contributors to simulation inconsistency is not knowing where the supplies are or finding them disorganized and incomplete. Your kit should live in a dedicated, clearly labelled space that is:

- *Easily accessible:* (e.g. a bin in the staff room or a shelf in a designated cupboard)

- *Clearly labelled* as "Simulation Supplies" or "Training Use Only"

- *Separate from clinical inventory*, especially when it includes medication containers, oxygen masks, or airway devices

Implement a Kit Checklist

Create a master "Simulation Kit Inventory Checklist" and include a printed copy inside your storage container. This should list all included items, quantities, and the last time they were checked or updated.
Encourage the facilitator or simulation lead to use the checklist:

- *Before each drill*: Confirm that the kit is complete and the props are functional.

- *After each drill*: Ensure all items are returned and

note any damaged or missing components.

- *Quarterly or biannually*: Conduct a more thorough review and refresh of the entire kit.

Label Clearly and Permanently

To avoid clinical confusion or misuse, every item in your simulation kit should be labelled: "TRAINING ONLY, NOT FOR CLINICAL USE"

- Include colour-coded tape, large printed stickers, or laminated tags for added visibility.

- Label the outside of medication bottles, epinephrine trainers, oxygen delivery tools, and mannequin accessories.

If repurposing any clinical items, use bold labelling to prevent them from being returned to active stock.

Assign a Simulation Coordinator

Appointing a staff member (such as a dental assistant, office manager, or hygiene team leader) to be the Simulation Coordinator can ensure continuity. Their role includes:

- Maintaining the simulation kit

- Tracking usage and inventory

- Leading or supporting monthly drills

- Reporting any issues or missing components

This responsibility can be rotated quarterly or annually if preferred, but having an identified point person helps prevent gaps in readiness.

Keep It Clean and Hygienic

Although simulation isn't clinical care, infection control still matters—especially when mannequins, masks, or reusable props come into contact with staff hands or faces.

- Disinfect reusable surfaces (mannequin faces, oxygen masks) after each use

- Avoid using real liquids in fake medications or glucose paste to prevent mould or spoilage

- Store all moulage makeup and accessories in sealed containers to prevent contamination or spills

Review and Refresh Annually

Once a year, perhaps during a slower season or tied to your office's emergency training review, plan a dedicated simulation kit check-up. During this review:

- Discard damaged, outdated, or uncleanable items and old makeup

- Replace missing labels or broken components

- Consider adding new props or upgrades if your budget allows

- Reprint or refresh laminated charts, symptom

labels, and scenario cards

This helps ensure the kit remains a reliable and trusted tool, rather than an afterthought gathering dust in a corner.

A well-maintained simulation kit signals a strong safety culture in your dental office. It empowers your team to respond confidently and calmly in the face of real emergencies—and supports your goal of making monthly simulation a sustainable, high-impact routine.

Optional Upgrades for Enhanced Training

Once your team is consistently running monthly simulations with the essential kit, you may wish to enhance your training experience with a few select upgrades. These tools can increase realism, deepen immersion, and provide additional layers of clinical decision-making, but they are not required to run meaningful and effective scenarios.

For many offices, these items are best added incrementally, based on interest, budget, and team engagement. The key is to build confidence and routine with simple tools first, then selectively enhance fidelity in areas where it will have the most training value.

High-Fidelity Mannequins

Advanced simulation mannequins can feature realistic skin texture, reactive pupils, chest rise, or electronic feedback on compressions and ventilations. These can be impressive and immersive, especially for airway, cardiac, or seizure scenarios.

However, they come at a significant cost and may require technical support or storage space. For most dental practices, they are a "nice to have" rather than a need. Many offices find that their existing CPR mannequins, used creatively, are sufficient for all simulated emergencies.

Bluetooth Speaker for Ambient Sounds

For some groups, adding auditory cues can dramatically increase the emotional fidelity of a scenario. A small Bluetooth speaker can be used to:

- Play laboured breathing for asthma or anaphylaxis cases.

- Simulate cardiac monitor alarms or oxygen saturation tones.

- Add ambient stressors like sirens or background noise.

Free or low-cost apps and online sound clips can be queued from a smartphone or tablet to enhance immersion without adding visual clutter or complex equipment.

Realistic Medication Trainer Devices

Upgrading from mock labels to purpose-built trainer devices can improve psychomotor accuracy and increase participant confidence.
Examples include:

- *EpiPen Trainer Devices* – Designed to mimic the

feel and operation of real auto-injectors without a needle.

- *Glucagon Kits (Trainer Versions)* – Allow teams to practice reconstituting and administering a simulated dose.

These items are especially valuable for reinforcing time-critical tasks that participants may rarely practice in real life but must perform flawlessly in an emergency.

Pulse Oximeter or Glucometer (Training/Demo Mode)

Where feasible, include functional (but non-invasive) tools such as:

- *Pulse oximeters* – Cheap, portable, and instantly familiar. These can be used to simulate desaturation in respiratory scenarios (or with a simulated readout prepared ahead of time).

- *Glucometers* – Can be used with dummy test strips or paper result cards to simulate hypo- or hyperglycemia readings.

These tools reinforce clinical assessment behaviour, prompting learners to gather objective data and make decisions based on findings, not just scenario cues.

Start Small, Scale Smart

These enhancements can elevate your simulation training, but they are not essential to building team readiness. Many dental offices run highly effective scenarios using just a mannequin, a timer, and a handful of well-labelled props.

Focus first on establishing a reliable monthly practice and a culture of psychological safety and team learning. Once that routine is in place, you can confidently and selectively invest in upgrades that serve your team's specific goals.

The Simulations

- The Syncope Simulations
- The Seizure Simulations
- The Diabetic Emergencies
- The Adrenal Crisis Simulations
- The Anaphylaxis Simulations
- The Stroke Simulations
- The Angina and MI Simulations
- The Hyperventilation Simulations
- The Asthma Simulations
- The Cardiac Arrest Simulations

The Syncope Simulations

Syncope- commonly referred to as fainting—is the most frequent medical emergency encountered in the dental office.[3] While often benign and self-limiting, syncope can be frightening for both patients and staff, and in rare cases, may signal or precipitate more serious underlying medical conditions such as cardiac arrhythmias or hypoglycemia. Its sudden onset, potential for injury, and overlap with other life-threatening presentations make it a critical condition for dental professionals to recognize and manage promptly.

In the context of dental practice, syncope is often triggered by anxiety, pain, the sight of blood or needles, or prolonged upright positioning, especially in younger or vasovagal-prone individuals. Elderly patients, on the other hand, may experience syncope from orthostatic hypotension, cardiac causes, or medication effects. Regardless of the etiology, a timely and appropriate response can prevent complications such as hypoxic injury, aspiration, or escalation to full cardiac arrest.

Why Include Syncope in Simulation Training?

Syncope presents a unique training opportunity: it is common enough to warrant routine preparedness but varied enough in presentation and underlying cause to require thoughtful assessment. Including syncope scenarios in simulation-based training supports several key educational goals:

Rapid Assessment and Differential Diagnosis: Is the patient simply vasovagal, or is this hypoglycemia, seizure, or even sudden cardiac arrest? Simulations encourage providers to think critically and avoid cognitive shortcuts.

Team Coordination Under Low-to-Moderate Acuity Pressure: Syncope scenarios enable teams to practice structured responses and role delegation without the intensity of a full-code situation, making them particularly useful for foundational team training.

Safe Patient Positioning and Monitoring: Dental chairs, physical layout, and the use of real equipment during in-situ simulation reinforce muscle memory for positioning the patient supine, administering oxygen, and preparing for escalation if needed.

Practice in Communicating With the Patient and Support Persons: Syncope is often reversible within minutes, and teams must be prepared to provide calm reassurance, obtain a relevant history, and make disposition decisions (e.g. resume treatment, reschedule, or refer).

Including syncope in your emergency training repertoire

ensures that staff are not only confident in recognizing and managing fainting episodes but also skilled in discriminating them from more serious emergencies, escalating care appropriately, and debriefing effectively after an event.

This chapter presents a range of realistic syncope simulation scenarios, each designed to emphasize clinical reasoning, communication, and team-based care in the dental setting.

Fainting After Needle Removal

Overview

A middle-aged woman faints moments after the completion of a local anaesthetic injection. The team must act quickly to manage vasovagal syncope and differentiate it from other causes of altered consciousness.

Learning Objectives

- Identify vasovagal syncope following procedural anxiety or stimulation
- Position the patient for optimal perfusion and airway safety
- Monitor and document post-syncope recovery
- Review considerations for rescheduling care or transport

Setup

Use a dental chair and simulate a local anaesthetic procedure. A participant can act as the patient, showing anxiety. Lay the chair back quickly to simulate intervention. Include a BP cuff, oxygen mask, and pulse oximeter.

Clinical Scenario (Narrative)

You've just completed a painless mandibular block on a 47-year-old woman scheduled for crown work. She appears relieved but then says, "I feel really hot..." and slumps in the chair.

Patient Presentation

Parameter	Value
Age/Sex	47F
Chief Complaint	Feeling hot and dizzy
Onset	Within 1 minute of injection
Vitals	HR: 55, BP: 84/56, RR: 14, SpO$_2$: 98%, Temp: 36.4°C
LOC	Briefly unresponsive (20 seconds)
Physical Findings	Pale, sweating, limp in chair

Clinical Course / Timeline

- **0 min:** Patient faints, becomes unresponsive
- **1–2 min:** Recovers consciousness slowly
- **3–5 min:** HR and BP gradually return to baseline
- **10 min:** Fully alert and stable

Critical Actions

- Recline chair, elevate legs
- Assess airway, breathing, and circulation
- Monitor vitals every 2 minutes until recovery
- Provide reassurance and observe for recurrence
- Document incident; consider postponing treatment

Discussion Questions

- How would you differentiate syncope from hypoglycemia or seizure?
- When should EMS be activated?
- What are the best practices for preventing vasovagal responses in future appointments?

Facilitator Notes (Optional)

- Learners may misattribute the collapse to an allergic reaction—redirect with clear vital signs.
- Emphasize prevention (patient positioning, conversation, stress management).

Syncope in the Waiting Room

Overview

A young adult becomes faint while waiting for her appointment. The scenario emphasizes the importance of early intervention in non-treatment areas and the need for staff-wide readiness in emergency situations.

Learning Objectives

- Recognize presyncopal signs before a procedure begins
- Apply emergency protocols in non-clinical areas
- Delegate tasks effectively in a team response

Setup

Set up a waiting area with a chair and a clipboard. Have a staff member or learner act as the patient. Use basic vitals equipment and simulate the arrival of the dental team.

Clinical Scenario (Narrative)

A 23-year-old woman is in the waiting room, visibly anxious about her upcoming root canal. As the assistant approaches her with intake forms, she says, "I don't feel so well," and collapses onto the floor.

Patient Presentation

Parameter	Value
Age/Sex	23F
Chief Complaint	Lightheadedness
Onset	Sudden, while sitting
Vitals	HR: 60, BP: 86/58, RR: 16, SpO$_2$: 99%
LOC	Unresponsive for 15 seconds
Physical Findings	Pale, breathing, regains consciousness on recline

Clinical Course / Timeline

- **0 min:** Patient collapses; staff responds
- **1–3 min:** Consciousness returns
- **5 min:** Moved to dental chair for monitoring
- **10 min:** Fully alert, anxious, refuses treatment

Critical Actions

- Call for the clinical support team
- Lay patient supine with legs elevated
- Monitor vitals, ensure airway patency
- Document and assess whether to continue care or refer
- Reassure the patient and provide water/snacks if recovered

Discussion Questions

- How do you modify your emergency protocol for incidents outside the operatory?
- How can dental teams prepare non-clinical staff for recognizing emergencies?
- What follow-up steps are appropriate when a patient refuses care?

Facilitator Notes (Optional)

- If learners leave the patient seated upright, simulate continued hypotension
- Debrief on risk management and staff roles

Syncope After Impression Taking

Overview

This case simulates syncope related to gagging during dental impression procedures, illustrating a physical stimulus as a trigger for a vasovagal response.

Learning Objectives

- Recognize reflex syncope caused by gagging or discomfort
- Perform airway repositioning and oxygenation if needed
- Document and manage the gag reflex to prevent recurrence

Setup

Use alginate impression trays and simulate a dental procedure with a seated patient. One learner acts as the patient, mimicking gagging and slumping. Use a BLS mannequin when practicing airway maneuvers.

Clinical Scenario (Narrative)

You are taking maxillary impressions on a 35-year-old male for whitening trays. The patient begins gagging, waves his hand, and then becomes pale and slumps forward in the chair.

Patient Presentation

Parameter	Value
Age/Sex	35M
Chief Complaint	Gagging, then fainting
Onset	Sudden, mid-procedure
Vitals	HR: 52, BP: 82/50, RR: 12, SpO_2: 95%
LOC	Brief unresponsiveness
Physical Findings	Gagging, sweating, limp posture

Clinical Course / Timeline

- **0–1 min:** Patient slumps forward, unresponsive
- **2–3 min:** Regains consciousness
- **5 min:** Vitals stabilize with positioning
- **10 min:** Patient reports nausea, unsure if they can continue

Critical Actions

- Stop the procedure and remove all instruments
- Reposition patient safely (supine with legs up)
- Ensure the airway is clear and breathing is adequate
- Provide oxygen and monitor vitals
- Reassess gag reflex management strategies

Discussion Questions

- How do gag reflex and vagal stimulation trigger syncope?
- What are safe airway interventions in a semi-conscious patient in the chair?
- What options exist to manage severe gag reflex in future procedures?

Facilitator Notes (Optional)

- If airway management is missed, simulate brief SpO_2 drop
- Encourage learners to reflect on how anxiety and discomfort interplay

Syncope During a Routine Dental Procedure

Overview

This simulation involves a young adult patient experiencing vasovagal syncope during a routine dental procedure. The case challenges learners to rapidly recognize the signs of syncope, initiate appropriate positioning and airway management, monitor vitals, and reassure the patient post-episode. It also reinforces the importance of team communication and prevention strategies in dental settings.

Learning Objectives

- Recognize early signs and triggers of vasovagal syncope in a dental patient
- Initiate immediate management, including positioning and airway protection
- Monitor and document vital signs, ensuring patient safety post-event
- Communicate effectively within the dental team and with emergency services if needed

Setup

- Use a dental chair or regular recliner to simulate the operatory.
- Have one participant act as the patient, another as a dental assistant, and one as the dentist.
- Use basic equipment commonly found in most dental offices, including a blood pressure cuff, pulse

oximeter, oxygen mask, and an emergency medical kit with ammonia inhalants (if used in local practice).
- For added realism, use makeup or a moulage kit to simulate pallor or sweat.

Clinical Scenario (Narrative)

You are a general dentist performing a lower molar extraction on a healthy 19-year-old male patient. The patient appeared slightly anxious upon arrival. As you administer local anaesthesia, the patient suddenly says, "I feel dizzy…" and then becomes unresponsive in the chair.

Patient Presentation

Parameter	Value
Age/Sex	19M
Chief Complaint	Fainting sensation
Onset	Sudden, during injection
Vitals	HR: 50, BP: 80/60, RR: 12, SpO$_2$: 98%, Temp: 36.5°C
LOC	Unresponsive, then responsive after 30 seconds
Physical Findings	Pale, diaphoretic, cool extremities, shallow breathing

Clinical Course / Timeline

- **Initial (0 min):** Patient reports lightheadedness and then slumps in the chair, eyes closed
- **1–2 min:** Patient remains unresponsive for 30–45 seconds, shallow breathing
- **3–5 min:** Patient regains consciousness, confused but improving
- **5–10 min:** Vitals normalize slowly, patient remains weak
- **10–15 min:** Full recovery with supportive care

Critical Actions

- Recognize syncope and call for help
- Recline the chair fully, elevate legs (Trendelenburg or supine with legs elevated)
- Open the airway and assess breathing
- Apply a pulse oximeter and monitor vital signs
- Provide oxygen if needed
- Reassure the patient post-event and monitor for recurrence
- Document the incident and discuss the need for further care or transport

Discussion Questions

- What are the common triggers of syncope in dental settings?
- What immediate positioning is most effective in this case?
- How would you differentiate this from other causes of loss of consciousness (e.g. hypoglycemia, seizure)?
- When would you consider activating EMS?
- What prevention strategies could reduce the risk of recurrence in anxious patients?

Facilitator Notes (Optional)

- If learners do not recline the patient quickly, prompt worsening vitals.
- If the airway is ignored, simulate brief desaturation (SpO_2 drops to 90%).
- Emphasize the importance of post-incident monitoring and documentation.
- Reinforce non-pharmacologic anxiety management strategies during debrief.

Repeat Syncope in a Known Fainter

Overview

A teenage patient with a history of fainting episodes begins to feel dizzy before anaesthetic administration. The focus is on anticipatory care, patient communication, and preventive positioning.

Learning Objectives

- Prevent syncope in a known at-risk patient
- Use positioning and calm reassurance effectively
- Recognize pre-syncopal cues and act early

Setup

Simulate an exam or local anaesthetic setup. Have the "patient" notify the team of feeling dizzy. Use a pulse oximeter and oxygen delivery devices as visual aids.

Clinical Scenario (Narrative)

You are preparing to extract premolars on a 16-year-old male with a history of fainting at the sight of needles. As you prepare the syringe, he says, "I think it's happening again…"

Patient Presentation

Parameter	Value
Age/Sex	16M
Chief Complaint	Lightheadedness
Onset	During anaesthetic prep
Vitals	HR: 58, BP: 88/60, RR: 14, SpO$_2$: 97%
LOC	Near-syncope only
Physical Findings	Pale, cool, clammy, seated upright

Clinical Course / Timeline

- **0–1 min:** Patient reports presyncopal symptoms
- **1–3 min:** Reclined early, avoids loss of consciousness
- **5 min:** Symptoms resolve with reassurance
- **10 min:** Patient calm, ready to proceed or reschedule

Critical Actions

- Identify pre-syncopal symptoms and respond early
- Recline the patient before loss of consciousness occurs
- Calmly reassure and engage in non-medical conversation
- Monitor vitals and document the event
- Decide collaboratively whether to proceed or defer care

Discussion Questions

- What are strategies to manage needle phobia or a fainting history?
- How can staff proactively reduce risk in these patients?
- What tools (verbal or procedural) help reduce anxiety-induced vasovagal response?

Facilitator Notes (Optional)

- If early action is not taken, simulate a loss of consciousness
- Highlight the importance of pre-treatment interviews and anxiety screening

The Seizure
Simulations

Seizures are sudden, uncontrolled electrical disturbances in the brain that can cause a wide range of symptoms, from brief lapses in awareness to full-body convulsions and loss of consciousness. In the dental office, seizures can occur with little or no warning and may be triggered by stress, pain, flashing lights, or interactions with medications. While many patients with a known seizure disorder will have a history and may be well-controlled, first-time seizures or breakthrough episodes remain possible and potentially dangerous.[4]

The dental setting presents unique challenges when a seizure occurs: the patient may be in a chair, under sedation, or holding sharp instruments in their mouth. Quick, composed action is essential to protect the patient from injury, support the airway, and monitor for prolonged or postictal complications. Dental professionals must recognize the signs of seizure activity, understand when to intervene, and know when to activate emergency medical services (EMS).

Why Include Seizures in Simulation Training?

Seizures represent a moderate-frequency, high-stakes emergency in dental practice. Though many episodes resolve on their own, they can escalate into prolonged seizures (status epilepticus), compromise the airway, or reveal an underlying undiagnosed medical condition. Training with seizure simulations enables the team to:

- Respond effectively, prioritize patient safety, and collaborate efficiently under stress.
- Improves Recognition of Seizure Phases and Presentations. Simulations allow providers to practice identifying both convulsive (tonic-clonic) and non-convulsive (absence or focal) seizures, including the often confusing postictal phase when patients may be disoriented or unresponsive.
- Reinforces Safe Chairside Management.
  Teams learn to clear the area of hazards, support the patient's head and limbs, and avoid inappropriate actions, such as trying to restrain the patient or inserting objects into the mouth.
- Strengthens Airway and Post-Seizure Monitoring Skills.
  Following a seizure, teams must assess airway patency, breathing adequacy, and vital signs, and determine whether the patient requires EMS transport, ongoing monitoring, or a family escort.

By preparing for seizure events through realistic simulation scenarios, dental teams can provide safer, more responsive care to patients with seizure disorders or unknown risk. The following cases will challenge your team to recognize seizures early, manage them confidently, and coordinate a patient-centred response in a calm, effective manner.

Seizure During Local Anaesthetic Injection

Overview

A healthy young adult experiences a generalized tonic-clonic seizure moments after receiving a local anaesthetic injection during a routine procedure.

Learning Objectives

- Recognize signs of a generalized tonic-clonic seizure
- Safely manage a seizing patient in the dental chair
- Identify potential causes, including anaesthetic toxicity
- Provide appropriate post-ictal care and reassurance

Setup

Use a mannequin or volunteer to simulate the seizure using limb tremors and altered consciousness. The dental chair should be set up mid-procedure with instruments visible. Use a sound clip or actor to simulate seizure sounds.

Clinical Scenario (Narrative)

You are midway through a dental filling on a 28-year-old male patient. You just administered 2% lidocaine with epinephrine. Suddenly, the patient stiffens, then begins jerking violently in the chair. An assistant yells, "I think he's having a seizure!"

Patient Presentation

Parameter	Value
Age/Sex	28M
Chief Complaint	None – mid-procedure
Onset	Sudden, during injection
Vitals	HR: 96, BP: 132/84, RR: irregular, SpO$_2$: 92%
LOC	Unresponsive during seizure
Physical Findings	Generalized jerking, frothing, clenched jaw

Clinical Course / Timeline

- **0 min**: Onset of seizure
- **2 min**: Jerking stops, patient remains unresponsive
- **5 min**: Post-ictal confusion, slow response to voice
- **10 min**: Vitals stabilize, patient groggy but alert

Critical Actions

- Stop procedure, lower the dental chair to a safe position
- Clear the area around the patient to prevent injury
- Do not place anything in the mouth
- Time seizure duration
- Monitor airway, breathing, and vitals
- Call EMS if seizure >5 minutes or first-time event
- Provide oxygen if SpO$_2$ <94%

Discussion Questions

- What signs suggest this was a tonic-clonic seizure?
- What local anaesthetic doses are considered safe?
- When should you call EMS during or after a seizure?
- What post-event documentation is required?

Facilitator Notes (Optional)

- If learners do not time the seizure, prompt them after 1 minute.
- If the airway is ignored, introduce desaturation on the monitor.
- Reinforce correct lateral positioning post-seizure.

Pediatric Febrile Seizure in the Waiting Room

Overview

A child in the waiting room collapses and begins seizing, unrelated to dental treatment. Office staff must respond quickly.

Learning Objectives

- Recognize febrile seizure presentation
- Perform pediatric BLS and seizure safety protocols
- Communicate effectively with caregivers and EMS

Setup

Use a pediatric mannequin or a small volunteer with a blanket. Place a thermometer, the child's chart, and a simulated parent actor nearby.

Clinical Scenario (Narrative)

A 4-year-old boy waiting for his first dental visit suddenly stiffens and begins jerking on the floor. His mother screams, "He's never done this before!"

Patient Presentation

Parameter	Value
Age/Sex	4M
Chief Complaint	Seizure in the waiting room
Onset	Sudden, witnessed
Vitals	HR: 118, BP: 96/60, Temp: 38.9°C, SpO$_2$: 97%
LOC	Unresponsive during the seizure
Physical Findings	Jerking limbs, flushed face, moist skin

Clinical Course / Timeline

- **0 min**: Seizure begins
- **1 min**: Child turns dusky, then improves
- **3 min**: Seizure stops spontaneously
- **5 min**: Crying, confused, mother tearful

Critical Actions

- Protect the child from injury (flat surface, padded)
- Do not restrain or insert anything in the mouth
- Monitor breathing and colour
- Record time and vital signs
- Contact EMS and reassure the caregiver
- Document fully and prepare to transfer care

Discussion Questions

- What features suggest this is a febrile seizure?
- How would your response differ for an afebrile seizure?
- What information should be relayed to EMS?

Facilitator Notes

- The parent actor can increase distress if learners don't provide reassurance.
- Introduce apnea briefly if no attention to breathing.
- Reinforce team communication during the emergency.

Status Epilepticus in a Patient on Phenytoin

Overview

A patient with poorly controlled epilepsy begins seizing in the operatory and does not stop after 5 minutes.

Learning Objectives

- Recognize and define status epilepticus
- Initiate emergency response and airway management
- Communicate with EMS clearly and efficiently

Setup

Simulate a prolonged seizure with an audio loop and a mannequin. Provide a patient chart that includes phenytoin in the medication list.

Clinical Scenario (Narrative)

A 60-year-old man is in the chair for a crown fitting. He stiffens, begins jerking, and the seizure continues beyond 5 minutes. His chart lists poorly controlled epilepsy and phenytoin.

Patient Presentation

Parameter	Value
Age/Sex	60M
Chief Complaint	Seizure
Onset	Sudden, prolonged
Vitals	HR: 110, BP: 150/90, RR: shallow, SpO_2: 89%
LOC	Seizing, no recovery
Physical Findings	Cyanosis, ongoing seizure

Clinical Course / Timeline

- **0 min**: Seizure begins
- **5 min**: No sign of stopping
- **7 min**: Cyanosis worsens
- **10 min**: EMS arrives

Critical Actions

- Recognize prolonged seizure >5 minutes
- Initiate emergency EMS call
- Maintain airway and provide oxygen
- Suction as needed
- Prepare handoff with history, medications, duration

Discussion Questions

- What defines status epilepticus?
- How do you support the airway of a seizing patient?
- What are the red flags for airway compromise?

Facilitator Notes

- If oxygen is not used, SpO_2 worsens.
- Prompt EMS call if not made within 5 minutes.
- Encourage rapid team role assignment.

Seizure Secondary to Hypoglycemia

Overview

A diabetic patient misses breakfast before an early appointment and seizes mid-procedure.

Learning Objectives

- Identify hypoglycemia as a seizure cause
- Administer glucose orally or via glucagon (if trained)
- Manage altered LOC and recovery

Setup

Place a glucose meter, juice box, and dental setup for a morning procedure. The patient's chart includes "Type 1 Diabetes."

Clinical Scenario (Narrative)

A 40-year-old woman with Type 1 diabetes arrives for a 9:00 am appointment. Midway through the procedure, she slumps, stiffens, and begins seizing.

Patient Presentation

Parameter	Value
Age/Sex	40F
Chief Complaint	Seizure
Onset	Mid-procedure
Vitals	HR: 98, BP: 110/78, RR: 18, SpO$_2$: 97%
LOC	Seizing
Physical Findings	Pale, sweating, clenching teeth

Clinical Course / Timeline

- **0 min**: Seizure begins
- **2 min**: Seizure ends
- **4 min**: Confused, unresponsive to voice
- **6 min**: Recovers partially after glucose gel

Critical Actions

- Protect the patient from injury
- Check glucose level if possible
- Administer glucose (oral or IV per scope)
- Call EMS if prolonged or unclear cause
- Monitor vitals, prepare for transfer

Discussion Questions

- What clues suggested hypoglycemia?
- What glucose sources are appropriate in the dental office?
- How do you document and follow up on such an event?

Facilitator Notes

- Provide meter reading if asked ("LO" or <2.0 mmol/L)
- Prompt glucose administration early
- Introduce repeat seizure if glucose is delayed

Seizure in a Known Epileptic Patient

Overview

A known epileptic patient seizes in the operatory during a cleaning visit. The team must manage a recurrent seizure and consider whether 911 is needed.

Learning Objectives

- Manage known seizure disorder in a dental setting
- Identify when emergency escalation is appropriate
- Reassure and communicate with the recovering patient

Setup

Use patient chart with "Hx: epilepsy" note. Simulate a seizure with audio and an assistant acting. Use a BP cuff and a pulse oximeter.

Clinical Scenario (Narrative)

A 35-year-old woman is undergoing a routine cleaning. She suddenly drops the suction, stiffens, and begins convulsing. Her chart notes a seizure history and daily medication.

Patient Presentation

Parameter	Value
Age/Sex	35F
Chief Complaint	None – mid-cleaning
Onset	Sudden
Vitals	HR: 104, BP: 138/84, SpO$_2$: 94%
LOC	Unresponsive, seizing
Physical Findings	Convulsions, clenched jaw, known epilepsy

Clinical Course / Timeline

- **0 min**: Seizure begins
- **2 min**: Spontaneous resolution
- **5 min**: Alert but confused
- **10 min**: Fully oriented, requests to rest

Critical Actions

- Protect from injury
- Time seizure duration
- Maintain open airway, monitor vitals
- Determine if EMS is needed based on seizure duration/recovery
- Document and debrief with the patient

Discussion Questions

- When is it safe not to call EMS in a seizure patient?
- How do you verify postictal recovery?
- How would you adapt future dental care for this patient?

Facilitator Notes

- If learners assume a first seizure, it introduces confusion over history.
- If the airway is ignored, simulate desaturation.
- Allow the patient to recover and ask questions to assess reassurance skills.

The Diabetic Emergency Simulations

Diabetic emergencies represent a critical, though often underappreciated, category of medical incidents that can occur in the dental office. With the global rise in diabetes mellitus—both type 1 and type 2—dental professionals are increasingly likely to encounter patients at risk of hypoglycemia, hyperglycemia, or diabetic ketoacidosis (DKA) during routine care.[3] These events may be triggered or exacerbated by missed meals, anxiety, medication timing, or the stress of a dental procedure.

Among these, hypoglycemia is by far the most common and urgent emergency, particularly in insulin-dependent patients or those taking oral hypoglycemics. Symptoms such as sweating, confusion, slurred speech, tremors, or altered responsiveness can occur rapidly and, if not recognized and treated promptly, may progress to seizures or unconsciousness. Conversely, while hyperglycemia and DKA are less likely to reach critical thresholds during a dental appointment, unrecognized signs (e.g. polyuria, fruity breath, fatigue) may indicate a serious underlying issue that requires prompt referral.

Why Include Diabetic Emergencies in Simulation Training?

Diabetic emergencies are often preventable with good patient screening and careful attention to timing, but they can still arise even in well-prepared clinics. Simulation training provides a unique opportunity for dental teams to practice both early recognition and a safe, coordinated response, thereby building confidence in managing these events.

Reactive Hypoglycemia After Local anaesthetic

Overview

An adult patient with type 2 diabetes becomes symptomatic after a lengthy procedure using epinephrine-containing anaesthetic.

Learning Objectives

- Recognize that symptoms of hypoglycemia and epinephrine toxicity overlap
- Distinguish between symptoms caused by hypoglycemia and those caused by epinephrine side effects from the anaesthetic, and respond appropriately
- Respond with appropriate monitoring and glucose

Setup

Simulate a patient in the chair with tremors and sweating. Provide a glucometer, juice box, and pulse oximeter.

Clinical Scenario (Narrative)

A 56-year-old female with type 2 diabetes has just completed a 90-minute crown prep under local anaesthesia. She says she feels jittery, weak, and nauseated. She skipped lunch due to the appointment.

Patient Presentation

Parameter	Value
Age/Sex	56F
Chief Complaint	Shaky, lightheaded
Onset	Immediately post-procedure
Vitals	HR: 108, BP: 130/82, RR: 20, SpO_2: 99%
LOC	Alert but anxious
Physical Findings	Diaphoretic, mild tremors

Clinical Course / Timeline

- **Initial:** Appears anxious, sweaty
- **3 min:** Complains of weakness and nausea
- **5 min:** Blood glucose is 3.1 mmol/L (56 mg/dL)
- **10 min:** Oral glucose given, symptoms resolve

Critical Actions

- Check glucose before attributing symptoms to anxiety
- Administer oral glucose
- Reassure the patient and monitor vitals
- Delay discharge until stable

Discussion Questions

- How can a local anaesthetic with epinephrine mimic hypoglycemia?
- What monitoring should be done post-op for diabetic patients?
- When is EMS warranted?

Facilitator Notes

- Encourage learners to distinguish sympathetic symptoms
- Ensure they don't overreact with inappropriate meds (e.g. beta blockers)
- In a diabetic patient, especially one who has fasted and undergone a stressful, prolonged procedure, reactive hypoglycemia is a real risk
- The dental team must check blood glucose before assuming the symptoms are due to anxiety or epinephrine, to avoid missing a dangerous hypoglycemic episode

Severe Hypoglycemia with Loss of Consciousness

Overview

An older diabetic patient becomes unconscious in the waiting room after arriving for a dental filling.

Learning Objectives

- Perform rapid assessment of an unresponsive diabetic patient
- Administer glucose gel or injectable glucagon
- Maintain airway and call EMS

Setup

Use a mannequin in the waiting area. Place the glucometer and the glucagon kit nearby. Use fake vomit or simulate aspiration risk to stress airway management.

Clinical Scenario (Narrative)

A 68-year-old male is found slumped in the waiting room. His wife says he didn't eat lunch yet and had taken his insulin. He is unresponsive and not responding to verbal stimuli.

Patient Presentation

Parameter	Value
Age/Sex	68M
Chief Complaint	Unresponsive
Onset	While seated in the waiting room
Vitals	HR: 58, BP: 100/60, RR: 10, SpO_2: 94%
LOC	GCS 9 (eyes 2, verbal 2, motor 5)
Physical Findings	Cool skin, shallow breathing, unarousable

Clinical Course / Timeline

- **Initial:** Unresponsive but breathing
- **3 min:** Blood glucose reads 1.9 mmol/L (34 mg/dL)
- **5 min:** Glucagon administered IM
- **10 min:** Regains partial consciousness

Critical Actions

- Conduct primary survey (ABC)
- Perform a glucose check
- Administer IM glucagon
- Position the patient laterally, monitor the airway
- Activate EMS

Discussion Questions

- What are contraindications to oral glucose?
- When and how is glucagon used in dental offices?
- How would you manage airway protection in this setting?

Facilitator Notes

- If the airway is neglected, simulate gurgling or cyanosis
- Reinforce the importance of lateral positioning

Hyperglycemia with Ketosis in a Teen

Overview

A teenager presenting for dental cleaning becomes progressively unwell due to undiagnosed type 1 diabetes.

Learning Objectives

- Recognize hyperglycemia and early DKA warning signs
- Identify red flags requiring EMS activation
- Support ABCs while awaiting transport

Setup

Use an actor with dry lips, flushed cheeks, and laboured breathing. Simulate acetone breath with nail polish remover nearby. Have a glucometer that reads "HI" or 28+ mmol/L.

Clinical Scenario (Narrative)

You're treating a 14-year-old female during a routine cleaning. She looks unwell and mentions nausea and "just feeling off." Her mother says she's been drinking water constantly and going to the bathroom frequently.

Patient Presentation

Parameter	Value
Age/Sex	14F
Chief Complaint	Nausea, fatigue
Onset	Began earlier that morning
Vitals	HR: 122, BP: 104/64, RR: 26, SpO$_2$: 97%, Temp: 37.5°C
LOC	Alert but fatigued
Physical Findings	Flushed skin, dry mouth, fruity breath

Clinical Course / Timeline

- **Initial:** Complains of nausea, appears flushed
- **5 min:** Reports abdominal pain and thirst
- **10 min:** Glucometer shows "HI" (>28 mmol/L)
- **15 min:** Develops deep, rapid (Kussmaul) breathing

Critical Actions

- Identify abnormal breathing and high blood sugar
- Place the patient in a comfortable position, monitor vitals
- Call EMS for transport and further care
- Reassure patient and parent, avoid oral fluids

Discussion Questions

- How does this presentation differ from hypoglycemia?
- Why is oral glucose contraindicated here?
- What signs point toward diabetic ketoacidosis?

Facilitator Notes

- If learners give sugar, introduce vomiting
- If no EMS is called, worsening LOC should be simulated

Hypoglycemia During Nitrous Oxide Sedation

Overview

A young diabetic patient under conscious sedation for a filling becomes confused and non-responsive to commands.

Learning Objectives

- Monitor blood sugar during sedation
- Identify altered LOC due to hypoglycemia vs oversedation
- Use oral/IV glucose appropriately and safely stop sedation

Setup

Use a nitrous mask, pulse oximeter, and sedation monitor props. Use an actor to appear drowsy/confused. Have glucose sources and EMS contact tools ready.

Clinical Scenario (Narrative)

You are using nitrous oxide for a 25-year-old type 1 diabetic during a lengthy filling. The patient becomes unusually quiet and does not respond to instructions. Your assistant notes he was shaking earlier.

Patient Presentation

Parameter	Value
Age/Sex	25M
Chief Complaint	Altered consciousness
Onset	30 minutes into procedure
Vitals	HR: 96, BP: 108/74, RR: 14, SpO$_2$: 98%
LOC	GCS 13, reduced responsiveness
Physical Findings	Clammy skin, sluggish speech

Clinical Course / Timeline

- **Initial:** Minimal response to voice
- **3 min:** Glucose reads 2.7 mmol/L (48 mg/dL)
- **5 min:** Procedure halted, glucose given
- **10 min:** Alertness returns, nitrous discontinued

Critical Actions

- Check glucose early in the sedation protocol
- Stop nitrous and provide oxygen
- Administer oral glucose
- Monitor closely and call EMS if no improvement

Discussion Questions

- How do you differentiate oversedation from hypoglycemia?
- What are the sedation protocols for diabetic patients?
- What if the patient becomes unconscious?

Facilitator Notes

- Encourage discussion on sedation risk screening
- Discuss fasting protocols and informed consent

Hypoglycemia in a Nervous Patient

Overview

A young patient with type 1 diabetes becomes hypoglycemic in the dental chair after skipping breakfast due to anxiety about an extraction.

Learning Objectives

- Recognize early signs of hypoglycemia
- Provide timely glucose replacement using office supplies
- Communicate effectively with the patient and family
- Know when to activate EMS

Setup

Use a mannequin or a live actor. Apply makeup for pallor and sweat. Place a glucometer and oral glucose on a tray. Have someone roleplay a worried parent or sibling.

Clinical Scenario (Narrative)

You are midway through a scheduled extraction for a 17-year-old male with type 1 diabetes. His mother mentions he was too anxious to eat this morning. Ten minutes into the procedure, he becomes pale, sweaty, and increasingly confused.

Patient Presentation

Parameter	Value
Age/Sex	17M
Chief Complaint	"I feel weird... dizzy..."
Onset	During procedure
Vitals	HR: 102, BP: 112/68, RR: 18, SpO$_2$: 98%
LOC	Drowsy, slow responses (GCS 14)
Physical Findings	Pale, diaphoretic, slurred speech

Clinical Course / Timeline

- **Initial:** Mild confusion, clammy skin
- **3 min:** Patient cannot respond appropriately to questions
- **5 min:** Blood glucose reads 2.4 mmol/L (43 mg/dL)
- **8 min:** Oral glucose administered
- **10 min:** Patient gradually improves

Critical Actions

- Stop the procedure immediately
- Perform a capillary glucose check
- Administer oral glucose or a sugary drink
- Monitor for improvement
- Prepare to call EMS if no rapid response

Discussion Questions

- How can you differentiate between anxiety and hypoglycemia?
- What are the most accessible glucose sources in a dental office?
- When is EMS activation necessary?

Facilitator Notes

- If learners skip the glucose check, the patient deteriorates
- If oral glucose is delayed, LOC may drop
- Reinforce that oral glucose is adequate if the patient is conscious

The Adrenal Crisis Simulations

Adrenal crisis is a rare but potentially life-threatening medical emergency that can occur in dental patients with adrenal insufficiency, such as those with Addison's disease or those on long-term corticosteroid therapy. While often overlooked, adrenal insufficiency becomes critically important during periods of physiological stress—such as dental surgery, pain, infection, or anxiety—when the body requires elevated cortisol levels. If the adrenal glands (or their synthetic replacement) cannot meet this demand, the patient may quickly decompensate.

An adrenal crisis can present with hypotension, weakness, vomiting, confusion, pallor, hypoglycemia, or loss of consciousness, and may be mistaken for more common conditions such as syncope, anxiety, or hypoglycemia. If unrecognized or untreated, adrenal crisis can progress rapidly to shock and death. Prompt administration of a corticosteroid (e.g. intramuscular hydrocortisone), fluid resuscitation, and EMS activation are critical interventions.

Why Include Adrenal Crisis in Simulation Training?

While adrenal crisis is not frequently encountered, it represents a high-risk, low-frequency event that requires immediate and coordinated action. Simulation provides an essential opportunity for dental teams to practice the rare but critical skills needed to recognize and manage this emergency effectively.

Although adrenal crisis is uncommon, its rapid onset, subtle early signs, and potentially fatal consequences make it an essential part of comprehensive dental emergency preparedness. The following simulation cases are designed to challenge your team's ability to identify at-risk patients, recognize early signs of crisis, and intervene with confidence and competence.

Child Collapse
An Adrenal Crisis in Pediatric Dentistry

Overview

A young patient with congenital adrenal hyperplasia (CAH) experiences a crisis after a stressful pediatric dental procedure.

Learning Objectives

- Recognize pediatric adrenal crisis presentation
- Communicate effectively with caregivers and EMS
- Apply pediatric BLS principles in an office setting

Setup

Child-sized mannequin or volunteer. Simulate a pediatric dental setting with a caregiver present. Include a mock emergency kit and oxygen.

Clinical Scenario (Narrative)

You're finishing a filling on a 7-year-old male with a known history of Congenital Adrenal Hyperplasia (CAH). He becomes flushed and lethargic in the chair. His mother reports he was due for a stress dose of hydrocortisone this morning but refused.

Patient Presentation

Parameter	Value
Age/Sex	7M
Chief Complaint	Sleepy, nausea
Onset	End of procedure
Vitals	HR: 128, BP: 78/42, RR: 30, SpO$_2$: 96%, Temp: 35.5°C
LOC	Responds to pain only
Physical Findings	Floppy, pale, dry mucosa

Clinical Course / Timeline

- **Initial contact**: Child sluggish, responsive
- **5 min**: Vomits and becomes less responsive
- **10 min**: Rapid pulse, hypotension worsens
- **15 min**: EMS arrives

Critical Actions

- Lay the child flat, elevate the legs
- Administer blow-by oxygen
- Prompt the caregiver to give hydrocortisone if available
- Call EMS and communicate the diagnosis and medication history

Discussion Questions

- How does adrenal crisis differ in children vs. adults?
- What role can caregivers play during emergency support?
- How can you adapt emergency kits for pediatric emergencies?

Facilitator Notes (Optional)

- Caregiver may offer oral or IM hydrocortisone — allow learners to facilitate that
- Reinforce pediatric BLS oxygen delivery and positioning

The Forgotten Steroid
A Post-Op Disaster

Overview

A patient on chronic steroid therapy for lupus fails to take pre-procedure stress dosing and experiences an adrenal crisis after a lengthy appointment.

Learning Objectives

- Understand the importance of perioperative steroid supplementation
- Recognize delayed adrenal crisis presentation
- Reinforce interprofessional collaboration with prescribing physicians

Setup

Simulate the post-op environment: the patient is in the waiting room or at check-out. The volunteer begins showing signs of collapse. Include mock prescriptions in chart notes.

Clinical Scenario (Narrative)

A 53-year-old female with lupus completes a 90-minute scaling and root planing appointment. While at the front desk, she feels faint and slides to the floor.

Patient Presentation

Parameter	Value
Age/Sex	53F
Chief Complaint	Fainting, fatigue
Onset	Shortly after procedure
Vitals	HR: 108, BP: 84/50, RR: 24, SpO$_2$: 93%
LOC	Responds to voice
Physical Findings	Flushed, slightly cyanotic lips, cool hands

Clinical Course / Timeline

- **Initial contact**: Patient weak and dizzy
- **5 min**: Begins vomiting
- **10 min**: BP drops to 70/40
- **15 min**: Loss of consciousness

Critical Actions

- Place patient supine, elevate legs
- Apply high-flow oxygen
- Call EMS and report lupus/steroid use
- Review the chart to identify missed stress dose
- Provide handoff to EMS with medication history

Discussion Questions

- What are common medications that suppress adrenal function?
- How can dentists coordinate with prescribers to avoid this scenario?
- What post-treatment observation protocols might help in high-risk patients?

Facilitator Notes (Optional)

- Consider having learners "discover" the missing steroid dose in chart notes
- Prompt discussion on stress-dose guidelines for dental procedures

Collapse During Crown Prep An Adrenal Crisis Unfolds

Overview

A known corticosteroid-dependent patient suddenly collapses mid-procedure, prompting rapid recognition of adrenal insufficiency and basic resuscitative interventions.

Learning Objectives

- Recognize signs and symptoms of adrenal crisis
- Initiate BLS-level interventions, including oxygen and positioning
- Activate EMS and communicate suspected adrenal insufficiency

Setup

Use a dental chair with a volunteer or mannequin. Have a dental assistant simulate a panicked response. Place mock oxygen equipment, emergency drug kit (with mock hydrocortisone), and a phone for EMS activation.

Clinical Scenario (Narrative)

You are midway through a crown prep on a 62-year-old male with a history of rheumatoid arthritis. He appears pale and suddenly slumps in the chair, unresponsive.

Patient Presentation

Parameter	Value
Age/Sex	62M
Chief Complaint	Unconsciousness
Onset	Sudden during procedure
Vitals	HR: 110, BP: 80/50, RR: 26, SpO$_2$: 94%, Temp: 35.8°C
LOC	Drowsy, responds to voice
Physical Findings	Diaphoretic, weak pulse, grey appearance

Clinical Course / Timeline

- **Initial contact**: Patient drowsy but responsive to voice
- **5 min**: Becomes unresponsive to verbal stimuli
- **10 min**: Vomiting begins, BP drops to 70/40
- **15 min**: EMS arrives if activated early

Critical Actions

- Position patient supine, elevate legs
- Apply oxygen via mask
- Ask the assistant to call EMS
- Retrieve emergency kit and consider giving IM hydrocortisone if trained and authorized
- Relay history of corticosteroid use to EMS

Discussion Questions

- What are typical triggers for adrenal crisis in dental settings?
- What should be communicated to EMS responders?
- How would management differ if the patient were on oral steroids vs. recent cessation?

Facilitator Notes (Optional)

- If learners hesitate to call EMS, introduce worsening hypotension and unresponsiveness
- If IM hydrocortisone is suggested, prompt discussion about scope and training

Routine Cleaning Gone Wrong – Adrenal Crisis in a High-Functioning Patient

Overview

A seemingly healthy patient experiences an adrenal crisis with no obvious signs of steroid dependence, requiring keen clinical suspicion and EMS involvement.

Learning Objectives

- Consider adrenal crisis in unexplained hypotension
- Emphasize communication and emergency team roles
- Reinforce oxygenation, positioning, and rapid EMS access

Setup

Use a dental chair, an assistant, and simple monitoring equipment. Provide a simulated incomplete medical history with vague "autoimmune disorder."

Clinical Scenario (Narrative)

A 60-year-old male, well-groomed and alert, comes in for a routine hygiene appointment. Near the end, he becomes dizzy, sweaty, and slurs his words.

Patient Presentation

Parameter	Value
Age/Sex	60M
Chief Complaint	Dizziness, confusion
Onset	Gradual end-of-visit
Vitals	HR: 118, BP: 82/46, RR: 24, SpO$_2$: 95%
LOC	Confused, slow speech
Physical Findings	Pale, diaphoretic, slumped posture

Clinical Course / Timeline

- **Initial contact**: Confused, diaphoretic
- **5 min**: BP continues to fall
- **10 min**: Nearly unresponsive
- **15 min**: Stabilization with EMS oxygen/fluids

Critical Actions

- Position patient, initiate oxygen
- Call EMS and report suspicion of adrenal crisis
- Re-interview the patient's spouse about autoimmune medications
- Prepare handoff to paramedics

Discussion Questions

- What are "hidden" risk factors for adrenal insufficiency?
- How would you handle uncertainty about diagnosis during an emergency?
- How can dental teams ensure effective communication during EMS handoff?

Facilitator Notes (Optional)

- Patient's spouse can volunteer key medication history mid-simulation
- If learners treat as vasovagal only, introduce hypotension progression

Missed Medical History

Overview

An anxious patient with a hidden history of Addison's disease becomes hypotensive during a routine extraction, prompting a need for rapid recognition and EMS activation.

Learning Objectives

- Identify subtle signs of adrenal crisis
- Practice thorough medical history-taking
- Reinforce the need for early EMS activation in hypotension

Setup

Simulated medical history form with missed "Addison's disease" entry. Dental operatory with standard equipment. Use a mannequin or participant to simulate collapse.

Clinical Scenario (Narrative)

A 47-year-old female presents for wisdom tooth extraction. She appears anxious but insists she's "fine." Shortly after local anaesthesia is given, she slumps forward and becomes confused.

Patient Presentation

Parameter	Value
Age/Sex	47F
Chief Complaint	Lightheaded, nausea
Onset	Gradual after the injection of anaesthesia
Vitals	HR: 124, BP: 76/40, RR: 28, SpO$_2$: 95%
LOC	Alert but confused
Physical Findings	Pale, nauseated, sweating

Clinical Course / Timeline

- **Initial contact**: Patient is dizzy and nauseated
- **5 min**: Confusion, BP drops further
- **10 min**: Unresponsive if untreated
- **15 min**: EMS arrival and stabilization

Critical Actions

- Stop the procedure immediately
- Lay the patient flat and elevate the legs
- Administer oxygen
- Review medical history for endocrine disorders
- Activate EMS

Discussion Questions

- What red flags were present before the crisis?
- How can offices improve history collection and flag high-risk patients?
- How does stress influence adrenal function in Addison's patients?

Facilitator Notes (Optional)

- Emphasize that local anaesthesia and procedural anxiety can be significant stressors
- Consider using a pre-filled medical history form with important clues omitted

The Anaphylaxis Simulations

Anaphylaxis is a rapidly progressing, potentially fatal medical emergency that can occur in any dental practice, often without warning. Although relatively rare, its severity and unpredictability make it one of the most critical conditions for dental teams to be prepared for.[5] Immediate recognition and prompt administration of intramuscular epinephrine can mean the difference between full recovery and serious complications, including airway obstruction, cardiovascular collapse, or death.

In a dental setting, anaphylaxis may result from exposure to common allergens such as local anaesthetics, latex, antibiotics, or preservatives in topical preparations. It can occur in new patients with no known allergy history or in patients who have previously tolerated a substance without issue. Early signs, such as skin flushing, rash, itching, or mild respiratory symptoms, can be subtle and are easily mistaken for anxiety or a mild reaction until progression becomes life-threatening.

Why Include Anaphylaxis in Simulation Training?

Because the treatment window is measured in minutes, and the signs of anaphylaxis can evolve quickly and unpredictably, simulation-based training is essential to ensuring dental teams can respond with confidence, coordination, and urgency.

In this chapter, you'll find simulation cases that span the spectrum from early recognition of mild allergic reactions to full-blown anaphylaxis requiring epinephrine, airway support, and transfer to emergency services. Each case is designed to reflect realistic challenges in the dental environment, promoting both technical and non-technical skill development.

By including anaphylaxis in your emergency training program, you are preparing your team to recognize and manage one of the most time-sensitive emergencies in outpatient care. Simulation scenarios ensure that every team member knows their role, trusts the protocol, and can act decisively before the condition progresses beyond control.

Delayed Anaphylaxis from Peanut Exposure

Overview

A patient eats a protein bar containing peanuts in the waiting room. During a long appointment, they develop delayed-onset anaphylaxis.

Learning Objectives

- Recognize delayed-onset food-induced anaphylaxis
- Identify the need for emergency medication and airway management
- Respond to evolving respiratory distress
- Coordinate with EMS and provide accurate event history

Setup

Place snack wrappers around the waiting area. Use an actor or mannequin in the chair who progressively deteriorates. Include a mock medication kit with epinephrine auto-injectors.

Clinical Scenario (Narrative)

A 35-year-old male attends a crown prep and eats a protein bar while waiting. Midway through the appointment, he becomes flushed and says, "I can't breathe right." You notice swelling in his neck and lips.

Patient Presentation

Parameter	Value
Age/Sex	35M
Chief Complaint	Trouble breathing
Onset	40 minutes after food intake
Vitals	HR: 125, BP: 82/48, RR: 30, SpO_2: 89%
LOC	Alert but gasping
Physical Findings	Neck swelling, audible wheeze, anxiety, urticaria

Clinical Course / Timeline

- **0 min**: Swelling and breathing difficulty reported
- **3–4 min**: BP drops further, cyanosis begins
- **6 min**: Stridor, possible airway obstruction
- **10+ min**: Improved if treated aggressively

Critical Actions

- Rapid IM epinephrine administration
- High-flow oxygen and patient positioning
- Immediate EMS activation
- Review and identify food allergy trigger
- Document signs and treatment timeline

Discussion Questions

- How does food-induced anaphylaxis differ in onset and progression?
- What role does patient history and intake documentation play?
- How would you handle a repeat exposure scenario?

Facilitator Notes

- Do not mention peanuts initially unless learners ask about recent food or activities. Encourage environmental awareness and history-taking.
- Describe symptoms worsening slowly to simulate delayed-onset anaphylaxis—e.g. "He's now coughing more and struggling to take a full breath."
- Ask how students would educate the patient and document an unreported peanut allergy or cross-contamination issue.

Anaphylaxis After Latex Exposure

Overview

A young adult presents for wisdom tooth extraction and has an undocumented latex allergy. Shortly after the staff members don gloves and begin the procedure, the patient reacts.

Learning Objectives

- Recognize non-medication triggers of anaphylaxis
- Identify and eliminate the source of allergen exposure
- Manage systemic allergic reactions appropriately
- Reinforce the importance of allergy history-taking

Setup

Use latex gloves as a visible prop if none of the participants have a latex allergy (non-latex alternatives are available for safety). Display hives on moulage or paper cutouts. Have a team member act out breathing difficulty.

Clinical Scenario (Narrative)

A 22-year-old female arrives for third molar extractions. Shortly after you insert the bite block and begin local infiltration, she reports itching hands and difficulty swallowing. You realize you used latex gloves.

Patient Presentation

Parameter	Value
Age/Sex	22F
Chief Complaint	Itching, trouble breathing
Onset	5 minutes after glove contact
Vitals	HR: 120, BP: 84/58, RR: 26, SpO_2: 91%
LOC	Alert but distressed
Physical Findings	Hives on face and arms, periorbital edema, inspiratory stridor

Clinical Course / Timeline

- **0 min**: Patient complains of itching and swelling
- **3 min**: Audible stridor and panic
- **6 min**: Cyanosis develops if untreated
- **10 min**: May become unresponsive
- **15+ min**: Responds to epinephrine, oxygen, and EMS arrival

Critical Actions

- Immediately remove the latex source
- Administer epinephrine IM
- Apply high-flow oxygen
- Position for airway protection
- Call EMS and document latex exposure
- Consider a second dose of epinephrine if there is

no improvement in 5–10 min

Discussion Questions

- What non-drug exposures can cause anaphylaxis in a dental setting?
- What are the signs of upper airway compromise?
- How would you document this incident for medical follow-up?

Facilitator Notes

- If learners overlook removing the allergen source (gloves), prompt with "You still have your gloves on."
- If participants miss stridor, describe progressively louder inspiratory sounds and voice changes.
- Some students may be reluctant to use epinephrine. Ask open-ended questions like: "What's your threshold for giving epinephrine when airway symptoms are present?"

Anaphylaxis After Local anaesthetic

Overview

A middle-aged patient receives a local anaesthetic injection before a routine filling and suddenly develops anaphylactic symptoms. The team must act quickly using emergency medications and manage airway and circulation until EMS arrives.

Learning Objectives

- Recognize early signs of anaphylaxis
- Administer epinephrine via intramuscular injection
- Manage the airway and provide oxygen support
- Coordinate emergency response and EMS activation

Setup

Use a dental chair with a CPR mannequin or actor. Apply moulage for facial swelling or hives. Use a mock auto-injector or practice syringe. Have a team member play the role of the panicked patient.

Clinical Scenario (Narrative)

During a routine restorative appointment, a 46-year-old male receives 2% lidocaine with epinephrine. Within minutes, he reports a scratchy throat and dizziness. You notice facial flushing and audible wheezing.

Patient Presentation

Parameter	Value
Age/Sex	46M
Chief Complaint	Throat tightness, dizziness
Onset	2 minutes post-injection
Vitals	HR: 112, BP: 90/60, RR: 24, SpO_2: 92%
LOC	Alert, slightly anxious
Physical Findings	Flushed face, mild lip swelling, wheezing, urticaria on neck

Clinical Course / Timeline

- **0 min**: Onset of symptoms after anaesthetic
- **3 min**: Lip swelling, wheezing increases
- **5 min**: BP drops further, patient reports feeling faint
- **8 min**: Loss of peripheral pulse, cyanosis if untreated
- **10+ min**: If treated early, the patient stabilizes with improved SpO_2 and BP

Critical Actions

- Recognize symptoms and call for help
- Administer 0.5 mg epinephrine IM (adult)
- Position the patient supine with legs elevated
- Administer high-flow oxygen
- Prepare a second epinephrine dose if needed
- Activate EMS and monitor vitals

Discussion Questions

- What are the key early signs of anaphylaxis in this case?
- Why is intramuscular epinephrine the first-line treatment?
- When would a second dose of epinephrine be indicated?
- How would you communicate this emergency to EMS?

Facilitator Notes

- If learners reach for antihistamines or salbutamol first, pause and ask: "Is this the first-line treatment for airway compromise and hypotension?"
- If learners delay giving epinephrine, cue deterioration: "The patient's BP is dropping. He looks pale and is slumping in the chair."
- If learners administer IM epinephrine early, reinforce by stabilizing vitals in real time.

Pediatric Anaphylaxis from Fluoride Varnish

Overview

A child in your office for a preventive visit receives fluoride varnish and quickly develops signs of a systemic allergic reaction.

Learning Objectives

- Recognize pediatric presentations of anaphylaxis
- Administer pediatric epinephrine dosing correctly
- Communicate effectively with guardians and EMS
- Provide psychological support while managing a crisis

Setup

Use a pediatric mannequin or child actor. Simulate facial swelling using cotton padding. Have a caregiver role-player present for realism.

Clinical Scenario (Narrative)

A 6-year-old boy receives topical fluoride varnish. Within minutes, he begins coughing, rubbing his eyes, and crying. His mother says he has a history of asthma but no known allergies.

Patient Presentation

Parameter	Value
Age/Sex	6M
Chief Complaint	Eye itching, cough, nausea
Onset	2 minutes post fluoride
Vitals	HR: 130, BP: 78/50, RR: 28, SpO_2: 93%
LOC	Crying, irritable
Physical Findings	Facial flushing, periorbital swelling, scattered wheezes

Clinical Course / Timeline

- **0 min**: Symptoms appear after the fluoride varnish
- **2–3 min**: Respiratory signs and anxiety increase
- **5 min**: Hypotension worsens
- **8 min**: If untreated, decreased LOC
- **12+ min**: Improves with IM epinephrine and oxygen

Critical Actions

- Recognize signs of pediatric anaphylaxis
- Administer epinephrine IM (0.15 mg for <30kg)
- Reassure and position the child safely
- Provide oxygen
- Involve the caregiver and call EMS
- Prepare for the second dose if needed

Discussion Questions

- How does pediatric anaphylaxis differ from adults?
- What barriers might prevent timely epinephrine use?
- How can dental offices prepare for child-specific emergencies?

Facilitator Notes

- Parental involvement: Use a standardized participant to play the parent. Ensure that learners explain what they are doing and obtain consent as they act.
- Ensure learners can identify the correct pediatric epinephrine dose (0.15 mg IM). If they hesitate, allow open-book reference or mock labels for the emergency kit.
- Introduce caregiver distress to simulate the stress of managing emergencies with a parent watching.
- Encourage learners to use age-appropriate and calming language for the child, even if they're acting on a mannequin.

Anaphylaxis from Antibiotic Premedication

Overview

A cardiac patient takes prophylactic amoxicillin in the office before a dental cleaning and experiences rapid-onset anaphylaxis.

Learning Objectives

- Understand the risks of antibiotic premedication
- Identify systemic allergic reaction signs
- Administer emergency medications
- Support airway and circulation until EMS arrives

Setup

Use a waiting room setup or chairside area. Use an actor to simulate collapse. Include a bottle marked "Amoxicillin" as a visual aid.

Clinical Scenario (Narrative)

A 70-year-old woman with a prosthetic valve takes amoxicillin 2g in-office before a periodontal cleaning. Fifteen minutes later, she feels nauseated, itchy, and unwell. She collapses while walking to the operatory.

Patient Presentation

Parameter	Value
Age/Sex	70F
Chief Complaint	Itching, nausea, lightheadedness
Onset	15 minutes post-antibiotic
Vitals	HR: 118, BP: 76/44, RR: 22, SpO$_2$: 90%
LOC	Semi-conscious
Physical Findings	Pale, clammy skin, audible wheezing, vomiting

Clinical Course / Timeline

- **0 min**: Sudden collapse in hallway
- **2–3 min**: Vomiting and airway compromise
- **5–6 min**: No improvement without intervention
- **10+ min**: Responds to epinephrine, oxygen, and EMS support

Critical Actions

- Administer IM epinephrine immediately
- Place the patient supine, elevate the legs
- Apply high-flow oxygen
- Monitor the airway for obstruction
- Call EMS and provide a handover on the medication timeline

Discussion Questions

- What key clues suggest anaphylaxis in this case?
- How would you differentiate anaphylaxis from vasovagal syncope?
- What is your documentation responsibility after such an event?

Facilitator Notes

- Ask whether they reviewed the patient's history and whether this allergy was previously documented.
- Use a training mannequin or actor who can "go limp" to prompt positioning and airway assessment.
- If symptoms persist after initial epinephrine, probe their knowledge on re-dosing intervals (usually 5–15 min).

The Stroke Simulations

Stroke is a time-sensitive, life-threatening medical emergency that can occur suddenly and without warning, even in the relatively controlled environment of a dental office. Although stroke is not caused by dental treatment itself, it may occur coincidentally during or shortly after a procedure, particularly in patients with predisposing risk factors such as hypertension, atrial fibrillation, diabetes, smoking, or a history of cerebrovascular disease. Because of this, dental professionals must be equipped to recognize the early signs and symptoms of stroke and activate emergency medical services without delay.

Recognizing stroke in the dental office can be especially challenging. Symptoms such as facial drooping, slurred speech, confusion, weakness, or coordination problems may be subtle at first or mistaken for fatigue, anxiety, or other less urgent conditions. In patients who are already reclined or have received local anaesthesia, small neurological changes can be easily overlooked.[6] The risk of delaying care, however, is significant—time lost is brain lost, and early recognition and EMS activation are essential to improving outcomes.

Why Include Stroke in Simulation Training?

Stroke scenarios are among the most critical components of a well-rounded emergency simulation curriculum. They reinforce the importance of early recognition, urgent action, and appropriate communication with emergency responders. Practicing stroke recognition and response in simulation helps dental teams refine their clinical vigilance, teamwork, and confidence in crisis communication.

By incorporating stroke simulations into your training, you prepare your team to act quickly and decisively in real-world situations where every minute counts. The following simulation scenarios are designed to reflect a variety of realistic presentations of stroke in the dental environment, from subtle early symptoms to dramatic neurological decline, helping your team practice safe, structured, and effective responses.

Delayed Recognition in a Busy Practice

Overview

A team is distracted by a full schedule and misses early signs of stroke in a patient recovering from sedation. The case emphasizes the importance of situational awareness and effective team communication.

Learning Objectives

- Identify subtle early stroke signs
- Maintain vigilance during post-op monitoring
- Coordinate team response under workload pressure
- Practice effective verbal handoffs and checklists

Setup

Use a recovery area or dental chair. Simulate multiple patients or noise. Use subtle actor cues (hand weakness, slight slurred speech) to challenge recognition.

Clinical Scenario (Narrative)

A 60-year-old woman is recovering from nitrous oxide sedation when she begins fumbling with her phone and slurring her words. A team member initially attributes this to lingering sedation.

Patient Presentation

Parameter	Value
Age/Sex	60F
Chief Complaint	Confusion, slurred speech
Onset	10 minutes after procedure
Vitals	HR: 82, BP: 158/90, RR: 17, SpO_2: 97%, Temp: 36.6°C
LOC	Alert, slightly drowsy
Physical Findings	Mild right-hand weakness, facial asymmetry

Clinical Course / Timeline

- **Initial**: Drowsy, uncoordinated
- **5 min**: Speech worsens
- **10 min**: Right leg shows mild weakness
- **15 min**: EMS arrives after stroke is recognized

Critical Actions

- Recognize stroke signs despite sedation background
- Confirm with neuro assessment and FAST
- Call 911 and give a clear report
- Maintain airway and monitor vitals
- Document onset and timeline

Discussion Questions

- How do you differentiate sedation effects from CVA?
- What systems can help avoid delayed recognition?
- How do you ensure smooth transitions and coverage during recovery?

Facilitator Notes

- Challenge learners to prioritize amidst distractions
- Reinforce checklists and observation protocols
- Reward early recognition with improved outcomes

Stroke Mimic: Hypoglycemia or CVA?

Overview

A diabetic patient presents with unilateral weakness and confusion. The dental team must decide if this is a stroke or a hypoglycemic event and respond appropriately.

Learning Objectives

- Recognize stroke vs. stroke mimics
- Perform basic differential assessment
- Administer oral glucose if indicated and safe
- Escalate care if symptoms persist after glucose

Setup

Use a dental operatory. Provide blood glucose reading tools (real or simulated). Role-play confused responses and one-sided body weakness.

Clinical Scenario (Narrative)

A 58-year-old diabetic male becomes confused and weak on the left side after receiving a local anaesthetic. He says he didn't eat this morning.

Patient Presentation

Parameter	Value
Age/Sex	58M
Chief Complaint	Weakness, confusion
Onset	Gradual over 10 minutes
Vitals	HR: 88, BP: 140/88, RR: 18, SpO$_2$: 97%, Temp: 36.7°C
LOC	Alert, disoriented
Physical Findings	Left arm weakness, slow speech, pale

Clinical Course / Timeline

- **Initial**: Disoriented, weak
- **5 min**: Glucose checked: 2.6 mmol/L (47 mg/dL)
- **10 min**: Oral glucose given, moderate improvement
- **15 min**: Still has some slurred speech

Critical Actions

- Check blood glucose if available
- Provide oral glucose or juice
- Call 911 if symptoms do not resolve
- Monitor vitals and LOC
- Document time and treatment response

Discussion Questions

- What signs suggested stroke vs. hypoglycemia?
- When is it safe to administer oral glucose?
- What would make you escalate to EMS?

Facilitator Notes

- If learners skip glucose check, delay symptom resolution
- If glucose is given and patient improves, reinforce mimic
- If no improvement, shift diagnosis toward stroke

Sudden Collapse in Reception

Overview

A patient in the waiting area collapses and becomes non-verbal. The dental team must differentiate stroke from other causes (e.g. syncope, seizure), perform a rapid assessment, and activate emergency procedures.

Learning Objectives

- Perform rapid neurological assessment
- Differentiate stroke from other collapse causes
- Maintain ABCs and ensure patient safety
- Coordinate roles and manage the scene efficiently

Setup

Use a chair or a waiting room setup. Place an actor or mannequin on the floor with one side immobile and simulate partial consciousness. Provide cue cards for team members.

Clinical Scenario (Narrative)

A 65-year-old male waiting for a crown prep collapses to the floor. He's breathing but unresponsive. His wife yells that he suddenly "stopped talking" and "slumped over."

Patient Presentation

Parameter	Value
Age/Sex	65M
Chief Complaint	Sudden collapse, aphasia
Onset	Sudden
Vitals	HR: 100, BP: 180/100, RR: 20, SpO$_2$: 95%, Temp: 36.8°C
LOC	Semi-alert, not responding verbally
Physical Findings	Gaze deviation, left-sided paralysis

Clinical Course / Timeline

- **Initial**: Collapse and aphasia
- **5 min**: Brief seizure-like twitching
- **10 min**: Slow improvement in responsiveness
- **15 min**: EMS arrival

Critical Actions

- Perform rapid neuro exam (AVPU, limb movement, gaze)
- Ensure an open airway and monitor breathing
- Document the last known normal and time of collapse
- Call 911 with a clear description of the event
- Clear the area and monitor the patient safely

Discussion Questions

- What signs indicate CVA rather than seizure or syncope?
- How does the patient's positioning affect management?
- What information will EMS need?
- How do you manage airway risks in this case?

Facilitator Notes

- Use gaze deviation or limb paralysis as key clues
- Prompt the team if they don't time/document the collapse onset
- Emphasize safety and scene control

Slurred Speech During Cleaning

Overview

A routine dental hygiene appointment is interrupted when the patient begins slurring their speech and showing signs of facial asymmetry. The team must recognize the stroke symptoms, initiate emergency protocols, and prepare for EMS handoff.

Learning Objectives

- Recognize signs and symptoms of an acute stroke (CVA)
- Initiate a stroke alert and call EMS promptly
- Support airway, breathing, and circulation while awaiting help
- Communicate clearly with emergency responders

Setup

Use a dental chair with a standardized patient (actor or mannequin). Apply makeup or stickers to mimic facial droop. Use scripted dialogue to simulate slurred speech and confusion, and include a clock to time the onset.

Clinical Scenario (Narrative)

During a routine cleaning, a 72-year-old female begins speaking unclearly. The hygienist notices her face seems uneven and alerts the dentist. The patient becomes confused and struggles to move her right arm.

Patient Presentation

Parameter	Value
Age/Sex	72F
Chief Complaint	Slurred speech, dizziness
Onset	Sudden, during the procedure
Vitals	HR: 84, BP: 162/94, RR: 18, SpO$_2$: 97%, Temp: 36.9°C
LOC	Alert, some confusion
Physical Findings	Facial droop (R), R-sided arm weakness, slurred speech

Clinical Course / Timeline

- **Initial**: Slurred speech, right-sided weakness
- **5 min**: Becomes increasingly confused
- **10 min**: Has difficulty following commands
- **15 min**: EMS arrival

Critical Actions

- Recognize FAST signs (Face, Arms, Speech, Time)
- Call 911 and document symptom onset
- Position the patient upright unless contraindicated
- Monitor vitals and prepare handoff report
- Reassure the patient and minimize movement

Discussion Questions

- What signs made you suspect a stroke?
- Why is it critical to note the time of symptom onset?
- What are your priorities while waiting for EMS?
- How would you handle airway concerns if LOC decreases?

Facilitator Notes

- If the team delays EMS call, simulate worsening symptoms
- Reinforce the importance of early stroke recognition and timing
- Provide positive reinforcement for calm team communication

CVA in the Dental Chair

Overview

Mid-procedure, a patient becomes unresponsive on one side and unable to speak. The team must safely stop the procedure and shift into emergency mode.

Learning Objectives

- Respond to stroke symptoms during active dental work
- Maintain patient safety during equipment removal
- Communicate effectively under pressure
- Prepare rapid EMS activation and an accurate report

Setup

Simulate a dental procedure in progress, including suction, instruments, and other equipment. Use a mannequin or actor with signs of facial droop and expressive aphasia.

Clinical Scenario (Narrative)

A 74-year-old man is midway through a crown prep when he suddenly stops responding and stares blankly. He is drooling from the right side and is unable to follow commands.

Patient Presentation

Parameter	Value
Age/Sex	74M
Chief Complaint	Sudden inability to respond
Onset	Instant during the procedure
Vitals	HR: 90, BP: 168/92, RR: 18, SpO$_2$: 96%, Temp: 37.0°C
LOC	Alert, nonverbal
Physical Findings	Right facial droop, right-sided hemiparesis

Clinical Course / Timeline

- **Initial**: Silent, slumped in chair
- **5 min**: Increased drooling, partial response
- **10 min**: Slight eye movement, no verbalization
- **15 min**: EMS arrives

Critical Actions

- Stop the dental procedure and secure the environment
- Position the patient upright or lateral
- Recognize stroke signs and call EMS
- Monitor vitals and airway
- Document time and clinical findings

Discussion Questions

- What are the signs of expressive aphasia?
- How do you safely transition from dental care to emergency response?
- How do you monitor for airway compromise?

Facilitator Notes

- If learners hesitate to stop the procedure, simulate worsening symptoms
- Prompt decision-making under pressure
- Reinforce safe positioning and communication

The Angina and Myocardial Infarction Simulations

Chest pain is one of the most alarming symptoms that can occur in a dental office. While many cases are benign—often related to anxiety or musculoskeletal tension—dental professionals must always treat angina and acute coronary syndromes (ACS), including myocardial infarction (MI or "heart attack"), as time-sensitive emergencies. These cardiac events are among the leading causes of morbidity and mortality worldwide, and they can present without warning in patients undergoing even routine dental care.

Certain dental procedures may increase stress or anxiety, potentially triggering angina or precipitating an infarction in vulnerable individuals. Risk factors such as hypertension, diabetes, smoking, obesity, high cholesterol, and a history of cardiac disease may increase the likelihood of an event. However, not all patients with cardiac ischemia will have a known history, which makes the ability to recognize symptoms and respond decisively critical.

Symptoms may include chest discomfort, shortness of breath, sweating, nausea, pain radiating to the jaw or arm, or an impending sense of doom. Dental professionals must be prepared to manage the situation promptly by stopping the procedure, administering oxygen and nitroglycerine (if indicated), monitoring vitals, and activating EMS without delay.

Why Include Angina and Heart Attack in Simulation Training?

Cardiac emergencies demand clear protocols, rapid action, and calm communication, all of which benefit significantly from simulation-based practice. Including angina and MI scenarios in simulation training prepares the dental team to intervene swiftly and potentially save a life.

Training for emergencies involving angina and MI:

- Promotes rapid recognition of cardiac symptoms. Simulation scenarios reinforce the importance of distinguishing true cardiac pain from anxiety or other non-cardiac causes. They help teams learn the typical and atypical signs of cardiac ischemia, especially in high-risk populations.
- Enhances Familiarity with emergency medications and protocols. Teams practice administering nitroglycerine, aspirin, and oxygen appropriately, while monitoring contraindications and side effects. Simulation also helps clarify when to activate EMS and how to communicate key details to responders.

By including angina and heart attack scenarios in your training program, you ensure your dental team is not only prepared to act but also to recognize and respond to cardiac events with clarity, confidence, and compassion.

The simulation cases that follow present a range of typical and atypical presentations, encouraging thorough, protocol-driven care in this high-stakes domain.

Silent MI in a Diabetic Patient

Overview

A diabetic patient with neuropathy reports unusual fatigue and jaw pain. The team must recognize non-classic MI signs and act swiftly.

Learning Objectives

- Recognize atypical MI symptoms in diabetics
- Use vital signs and history to guide care
- Practice full primary assessment with early EMS activation

Setup

- Dental operatory with routine procedure in progress
- Patient chart with history of diabetes and hypertension
- Include role-play for staff and EMS communication

Clinical Scenario (Narrative)

A 60-year-old female diabetic patient undergoing a hygiene visit reports jaw discomfort, fatigue, and lightheadedness. She denies chest pain but says she "just feels off."

Patient Presentation

Parameter	Value
Age/Sex	60F
Chief Complaint	Fatigue, jaw pain
Onset	15 minutes ago
Vitals	HR: 108, BP: 110/74, RR: 20, SpO_2: 95%, Temp: 37.0°C
LOC	Alert, slightly confused
Physical Findings	Sweaty, clutching jaw, cool hands

Clinical Course / Timeline

- **0 min:** Reports jaw pain and "feeling weird"
- **5 min:** Vital signs taken; HR elevated
- **10 min:** Appears pale, asks to lie down
- **15 min:** Becomes nauseated, HR rises to 120

Critical Actions

- Recognize atypical symptoms as potential MI
- Administer oxygen and aspirin
- Call 911 with diabetic history and jaw pain details
- Monitor vitals and LOC closely

Discussion Questions

- How does diabetes affect MI presentation?
- What clues differentiate this from anxiety or hypoglycemia?
- How can you avoid anchoring bias in diagnosis?

Facilitator Notes

- If hypoglycemia is considered, allow glucose test (normal)
- If aspirin is delayed, the patient deteriorates further

Angina in a Known Cardiac Patient

Overview

A long-term patient with known stable angina experiences chest discomfort during a procedure. The team must decide whether it is a routine event or something more ominous.

Learning Objectives

- Recognize changes from baseline angina symptoms
- Understand nitroglycerine use in a dental setting
- Practice decision-making under uncertainty

Setup

- Simulated patient with medical history on file
- Have a mock nitroglycerine spray and aspirin available
- Use a dental chair to simulate a mid-procedure setting

Clinical Scenario (Narrative)

A 71-year-old female with a history of angina reports mild chest discomfort after reclining for a filling. She has nitroglycerine spray in her purse and says, "This sometimes happens."

Patient Presentation

Parameter	Value
Age/Sex	71F
Chief Complaint	Chest tightness
Onset	2 minutes ago
Vitals	HR: 76, BP: 118/70, RR: 16, SpO$_2$: 99%, Temp: 36.8°C
LOC	Alert and oriented
Physical Findings	Calm, requesting her own nitroglycerine

Clinical Course / Timeline

- **0 min:** Reports discomfort, 3/10
- **5 min:** No relief after rest; wants to use nitroglycerine spray
- **8 min:** BP drops to 98/60 after nitroglycerine, pain 4/10
- **10 min:** Pain increases; she appears more anxious

Critical Actions

- Assess history and current symptoms thoroughly
- Confirm nitroglycerine dose and assist if within protocol
- Monitor vitals closely after nitroglycerine
- Call EMS if symptoms persist or worsen

Discussion Questions

- When is chest pain "different enough" to be considered emergent?
- Should you rely on the patient's self-assessment?
- When is EMS activation justified even for known angina?

Facilitator Notes

- Push learners to consider worsening symptoms and repeat nitroglycerine administration risks

Crushing Pain in the Waiting Room

Overview

A walk-in patient waiting for an urgent appointment collapses with crushing chest pain. The staff must act without prior patient records and manage a deteriorating condition.

Learning Objectives

- Perform primary assessment on an unknown patient
- Recognize signs of acute coronary syndrome (ACS)
- Deliver aspirin, oxygen, and EMS activation efficiently

Setup

- Use a waiting area chair and a staff member role-playing the patient
- Have a blood pressure cuff and oxygen mask available
- Include mock emergency medical forms and an EMS checklist

Clinical Scenario (Narrative)

A 59-year-old male presents for an emergency dental exam and begins experiencing severe chest pain. He slumps over, grimacing and clutching his chest. No medical history is available.

Patient Presentation

Parameter	Value
Age/Sex	59M
Chief Complaint	Severe chest pain
Onset	Sudden, 2 minutes ago
Vitals	HR: 102, BP: 132/86, RR: 22, SpO$_2$: 97%, Temp: 37.2°C
LOC	Alert but distressed
Physical Findings	Cool skin, sweating, visibly in pain

Clinical Course / Timeline

- **0 min:** Patient reports 9/10 crushing chest pain
- **3 min:** Reports radiation to jaw and left arm
- **8 min:** Begins to vomit, becomes pale
- **12 min:** BP drops to 90/58

Critical Actions

- Immediate call to EMS
- Administer aspirin (ensure not allergic)
- Provide oxygen
- Reassess vitals every 2–3 minutes
- Gather any medical alert bracelets or clues to history

Discussion Questions

- What are the red flags of myocardial infarction in undiagnosed patients?
- What are the risks if aspirin or EMS is delayed?

Facilitator Notes

- Encourage role-playing communication with EMS
- If learners hesitate, the patient's condition worsens (hypotension, vomiting)

MI in a Sedation Recovery Room

Overview

A post-IV sedation patient begins experiencing nausea and vague chest discomfort. Staff must differentiate sedation effects from cardiac signs.

Learning Objectives

- Recognize atypical signs of MI
- Understand post-procedural risk periods
- Coordinate EMS activation with airway monitoring

Setup

- Simulate the sedation recovery area
- Include monitors (real or simulated), oxygen delivery devices
- Use post-op documentation and vitals charts

Clinical Scenario (Narrative)

A 66-year-old male is recovering from IV sedation. He becomes pale, reports nausea, and describes a dull ache in the chest. He is breathing adequately but appears uncomfortable.

Patient Presentation

Parameter	Value
Age/Sex	66M
Chief Complaint	Nausea and chest ache
Onset	10 minutes post-procedure
Vitals	HR: 98, BP: 126/78, RR: 20, SpO$_2$: 96%, Temp: 36.6°C
LOC	Alert but sluggish
Physical Findings	Pale, mildly diaphoretic, holding chest lightly

Clinical Course / Timeline

- **0 min:** Mild chest ache, post-op
- **5 min:** Increases in discomfort, HR rises to 112
- **10 min:** Becomes diaphoretic, BP drops to 100/66
- **15 min:** Patient vomits and appears confused

Critical Actions

- Monitor ABCs, apply oxygen
- Administer aspirin
- Activate EMS
- Reassess every 3 minutes and prepare to hand off to EMS

Discussion Questions

- What makes MI easy to miss in sedation recovery?
- What vitals trends suggest worsening perfusion?
- Should you delay EMS activation to observe?

Facilitator Notes

- Increase realism with sedation paperwork, mock monitors
- Prompt on whether further sedation reversal is needed

Chest Pressure During a Crown Prep

Overview

A patient begins experiencing chest pressure and shortness of breath during a routine dental crown preparation. The team must recognize cardiac symptoms, provide immediate care, and activate EMS.

Learning Objectives

- Identify early signs of angina and myocardial infarction
- Administer aspirin and oxygen as per protocol
- Initiate EMS activation and maintain patient stability until arrival

Setup

- Use a dental chair with a patient actor or mannequin
- Simulate an operatory with typical dental tools, vital signs monitor (or simulated readouts)
- Role-play assistant and EMS contact

Clinical Scenario (Narrative)

During a routine crown preparation, a 63-year-old male reports chest pressure and "a heavy feeling" in his chest. He looks pale and is sweating. He mentions similar discomfort during yard work last week, but didn't see a doctor.

Patient Presentation

Parameter	Value
Age/Sex	63M
Chief Complaint	Chest pressure
Onset	Began 5 minutes ago
Vitals	HR: 88, BP: 142/88, RR: 18, SpO$_2$: 98%, Temp: 36.9°C
LOC	Alert and oriented (GCS 15)
Physical Findings	Diaphoretic, anxious, clutching chest

Clinical Course / Timeline

- **0 min:** Patient reports chest pressure
- **5 min:** Pain rated 7/10; becomes pale and diaphoretic
- **10 min:** Pain not relieved by rest; more anxious
- **15 min:** Reports nausea, BP drops to 100/60

Critical Actions

- Stop the dental procedure immediately
- Administer oxygen and chewable aspirin
- Call 911 and report cardiac symptoms
- Prepare for EMS handoff with vital signs and timeline

Discussion Questions

- How can you differentiate angina from MI?
- What is your scope in administering aspirin and oxygen?
- What information should you relay to EMS?

Facilitator Notes (Optional)

- If aspirin is delayed, the patient worsens
- Provide a mock 12-lead ECG readout if requested, showing nonspecific changes

The Hyperventilation Simulations

Hyperventilation is one of the most common anxiety-related medical events encountered in dental practice.[5] Though often benign, it can present with dramatic and alarming symptoms—chest pain, dizziness, shortness of breath, paresthesia, and even transient loss of consciousness—mimicking more serious conditions such as asthma, hypoglycemia, or cardiac events. Because of this, hyperventilation requires careful assessment, reassurance, and symptom management to avoid unnecessary escalation and ensure patient safety.

Hyperventilation typically occurs in response to procedural anxiety, phobia, or situational stress, particularly in patients with underlying anxiety disorders or poor coping strategies. It can be triggered before, during, or even after treatment. Dental professionals must be skilled not only in recognizing the signs and symptoms but also in differentiating hyperventilation from more dangerous pathologies that require emergency intervention.

Why Include Hyperventilation in Simulation Training?

Although not a life-threatening condition in most cases, hyperventilation can significantly disrupt patient care, provoke fear among staff, and—if mismanaged—result in adverse outcomes. Simulation-based training offers a controlled, realistic environment for teams to develop the confidence and judgment necessary to manage this scenario with calm and clarity.

A hyperventilation simulation:

- Supports the development of non-pharmacologic management skills. Effective responses to hyperventilation often require verbal reassurance, coaching in breathing techniques, and maintaining a calming presence. These are soft skills that improve with practice and reflection.

- Reinforces airway and oxygen use judgment. Learners gain experience in deciding when to avoid unnecessary oxygen use (which may heighten the patient's anxiety) and when to escalate if the patient's condition deteriorates.

Including hyperventilation scenarios in your simulation curriculum encourages a thoughtful, patient-centred approach to what is often a misunderstood emergency. The following cases provide realistic and varied presentations, emphasizing both clinical discernment and empathetic communication, to ensure your team is prepared to respond confidently and appropriately in the dental setting.

Teen with a Panic History

Overview

A teen patient with a history of panic attacks starts to hyperventilate during impression taking.

Learning Objectives

- Handle adolescent patients with known anxiety disorders
- Incorporate parental support effectively
- Use de-escalation techniques in physically awkward procedures

Setup

Use impression trays and alginate mix. Ask a parent to participate in scenario role-play.

Clinical Scenario (Narrative)

A 16-year-old is in the chair for orthodontic impressions. Midway through the upper tray placement, the patient gags and starts to panic.

Patient Presentation

Parameter	Value
Age/Sex	16M
Chief Complaint	"I can't breathe, I'm gonna choke"
Onset	During impression tray insertion
Vitals	HR: 104, BP: 130/82, RR: 34, SpO_2: 99%
LOC	Alert, scared, sobbing

Clinical Course / Timeline

- **Initial**: Panic and gagging
- **2 min**: Tray removed, breathing improves slightly
- **6 min**: Symptoms resolve with parent involvement

Critical Actions

- Remove physical trigger
- Involve parents for reassurance
- Guide slow breathing and offer rescheduling if needed

Discussion Questions

- What strategies work best with teens experiencing anxiety?
- How can you prevent gag reflex triggers?
- Should treatment be attempted again that day?

Facilitator Notes

- If learners attempt to continue with impressions, the patient may vomit
- Reinforce patient-centred care and psychological safety

Unexpected Panic During a Cleaning

Overview

A routine hygiene appointment is interrupted when an older patient suddenly becomes distressed and begins hyperventilating.

Learning Objectives

- Identify and manage panic attacks in older patients
- Recognize when symptoms may mimic cardiac or respiratory issues
- Communicate clearly with the patient and document appropriately

Setup

Simulate a hygiene station with ultrasonic scaler noise. Use a mock patient chart with a history of hypertension.

Clinical Scenario (Narrative)

A 62-year-old woman is receiving a routine cleaning when she begins clutching her chest and says she feels dizzy and breathless.

Patient Presentation

Parameter	Value
Age/Sex	62F
Chief Complaint	"My heart is racing, I can't breathe"
Onset	Sudden, during cleaning
Vitals	HR: 110, BP: 150/94, RR: 28, SpO$_2$: 97%
LOC	Alert, anxious
Physical Findings	Trembling, shallow breaths, perspiring lightly

Clinical Course / Timeline

- **Initial**: Symptoms suggest a cardiac or respiratory issue
- **5 min**: Reassurance leads to slowing of breathing
- **10 min**: HR and BP normalize

Critical Actions

- Reassure and take full vitals
- Rule out cardiac signs (pain radiation, ST changes)
- Guide deep breathing, avoid unnecessary oxygen
- Document episode and defer further treatment

Discussion Questions

- How can providers differentiate between cardiac and anxiety-related symptoms?
- What documentation is essential after such events?
- What if the patient insists on continuing treatment?

Facilitator Notes

- If learners give nitroglycerine, discuss the indications
- Use vague symptoms to encourage differential thinking

The Nervous New Patient

Overview

A young adult becomes increasingly anxious during the administration of local anaesthesia, leading to rapid breathing and signs of hyperventilation.

Learning Objectives

- Recognize early signs of hyperventilation due to anxiety
- Differentiate between anxiety-induced symptoms and medical emergencies
- Practice calming communication and non-pharmacological interventions

Setup

Use a standard dental chair setup. Have a team member simulate the patient. Use ambient background noise (e.g. drill sounds) and play out rising anxiety with verbal cues ("I don't feel right… I can't catch my breath").

Clinical Scenario (Narrative)

You are midway through preparing for a restorative procedure on a 22-year-old female. Moments after injecting local anaesthetic, she starts breathing rapidly, saying she feels dizzy and tingly.

Patient Presentation

Parameter	Value
Age/Sex	22F
Chief Complaint	"I feel lightheaded and my fingers are tingling"
Onset	Immediate, after LA injection
Vitals	HR: 102, BP: 128/84, RR: 32, SpO$_2$: 99%
LOC	Alert but panicked
Physical Findings	Pale, breathing rapidly, clenching hands, perioral numbness

Clinical Course / Timeline

- **Initial**: Anxious, breathing fast, vitals stable
- **3 min**: Reports chest tightness, lightheadedness increases
- **6 min**: Hand/finger spasm, tingling worsens
- **10 min**: With verbal reassurance and slowed breathing, symptoms resolve

Critical Actions

- Recognize symptoms as hyperventilation, not cardiac or allergic
- Guide the patient through slow, controlled breathing
- Reassure without offering oxygen

- Rule out anaphylaxis or local anaesthetic toxicity

Discussion Questions

- How can hyperventilation be differentiated from other emergencies?
- When should oxygen be withheld in this situation?
- What calming strategies can be applied during dental treatment?

Facilitator Notes

- If learners administer oxygen, prompt a review of when it's contraindicated
- Reinforce the importance of non-pharmacological de-escalation strategies

First Dental Visit in Years

Overview

An adult patient presenting for emergency dental care begins to hyperventilate while waiting for the freezing to take effect.

Learning Objectives

- Identify pre-procedural anxiety and hyperventilation
- Prevent escalation by addressing anxiety early
- Provide safe reassurance without overmedicalizing

Setup

Have a staff member act as the patient in a chair with topical anaesthetic in place. Dim lights to simulate a calming environment if de-escalation occurs.

Clinical Scenario (Narrative)

A 45-year-old man presents with dental pain after avoiding care for 10 years. After the local anaesthetic is administered, he becomes wide-eyed, breathing quickly, and states, "Something's not right…"

Patient Presentation

Parameter	Value
Age/Sex	45M
Chief Complaint	"I feel dizzy and can't breathe."
Onset	Just after the local anaesthetic injection
Vitals	HR: 106, BP: 142/86, RR: 30, SpO$_2$: 98%
LOC	Alert, mildly agitated
Physical Findings	Cold, clammy hands, dry mouth, fast breathing

Clinical Course / Timeline

- **Initial**: Appears to be reacting to the injection
- **3 min**: No rash, stable vitals suggest anxiety
- **7 min**: Deep breathing and distraction help calm the patient

Critical Actions

- Rule out allergic reaction or local anaesthetic toxicity
- Offer reassurance, distraction (music, conversation)
- Delay treatment briefly to allow calming
- Document and consider anxiolytic premedication for the next visit

Discussion Questions

- How can anxiety-related hyperventilation mimic an allergic reaction?
- What non-drug approaches reduce procedural anxiety?
- When is medical referral or postponement appropriate?

Facilitator Notes

- If learners initiate emergency medications, clarify assessment and reasoning
- Encourage discussion of pre-procedural planning for anxious patients

Claustrophobia in the Chair

Overview

A patient with a known history of claustrophobia begins to panic during radiographs, progressing to hyperventilation.

Learning Objectives

- Identify triggers and early signs of panic-related hyperventilation
- Apply distraction, verbal calming, and environmental control techniques
- Practice coordination between the assistant and the provider in response

Setup

Use X-ray bib and bitewing film placement as part of the scenario. Have the patient-actor resist and become visibly distressed.

Clinical Scenario (Narrative)

You are preparing to take bitewing radiographs on a 35-year-old male. As the X-ray bib is placed and the sensor inserted, the patient starts fidgeting, then begins breathing rapidly and says, "I need to get out of here."

Patient Presentation

Parameter	Value
Age/Sex	35M
Chief Complaint	"I feel like I can't breathe"
Onset	During X-ray setup
Vitals	HR: 98, BP: 140/90, RR: 30, SpO$_2$: 98%
LOC	Alert and anxious
Physical Findings	Rapid breathing, clutching bib, flushed face

Clinical Course / Timeline

- **Initial**: Mild panic, elevated respiratory rate
- **2 min**: Symptoms worsen with continued equipment use
- **5 min**: Symptoms resolve with repositioning and calm talking

Critical Actions

- Recognize claustrophobia and remove environmental triggers
- Calm patient and guide controlled breathing
- Avoid unnecessary medications or interventions

Discussion Questions

- How might the dental environment be modified to reduce patient anxiety?
- What role can the assistant play in de-escalating panic?
- When is it appropriate to reschedule treatment?

Facilitator Notes

- Introduce elevated vitals to simulate a sympathetic response
- Have the learner practice breathing techniques with the patient

The Asthma Simulations

Asthma is a common chronic respiratory condition that can become a serious, even life-threatening, emergency in the dental setting. Characterized by airway hyperresponsiveness, bronchospasm, and inflammation, asthma can be triggered or worsened by a number of stressors commonly encountered during dental visits, including anxiety, allergens (e.g. latex or disinfectants), respiratory infections, cold air, or even dental materials. Although most asthma attacks are mild and reversible with medication, severe exacerbations require rapid recognition and treatment to prevent respiratory failure.[7]

Dental patients with asthma may present with wheezing, coughing, shortness of breath, chest tightness, or difficulty speaking. In moderate to severe attacks, cyanosis, altered mental status, and silent chest (a lack of audible wheezing) may indicate critical airway obstruction. In such cases, dental professionals must act quickly to administer bronchodilators, monitor vital signs, position the patient appropriately, and activate EMS when necessary.

Why Include Asthma in Simulation Training?

Asthma is one of the most common chronic diseases globally, and dental teams are very likely to encounter patients with active or historical symptoms. Simulation-based training provides dental teams with the opportunity to prepare for a range of scenarios—from mild distress to near-fatal asthma attacks—so they can respond effectively and without hesitation.

Including asthma simulations in dental emergency training enhances team readiness for a common yet potentially life-threatening event. These scenarios encourage early recognition, confident use of medications, and clear communication skills that can make a critical difference when every breath counts.

Asthma Triggered by Dental Materials

Overview

A patient begins experiencing respiratory distress following exposure to strong dental disinfectants or bonding agents.

Learning Objectives

- Identify environmental asthma triggers in a dental clinic
- Take rapid action to remove the trigger and ventilate the area
- Support the patient until EMS arrives

Setup

Set up in an operatory with a "trigger" scenario (e.g. use a cotton roll scented with vinegar to simulate strong odours). Use fans to simulate ventilation efforts.

Clinical Scenario (Narrative)

A 45-year-old man with a mild asthma history is having a crown prep. Shortly after the bonding agent is applied, he begins coughing violently and reports chest tightness.

Patient Presentation

Parameter	Value
Age/Sex	45M
Chief Complaint	Shortness of breath
Onset	Immediate after bonding agent
Vitals	HR: 98, BP: 130/84, RR: 22, SpO_2: 95%
LOC	Alert
Physical Findings	Flushed, audible wheeze, mild tremors

Clinical Course / Timeline

- **0 min**: Initial coughing and mild SOB
- **5 min**: SpO_2 drops to 92%, audible wheezing
- **10 min**: Patient becomes increasingly panicked
- **15 min**: No response to one dose of the inhaler

Critical Actions

- Stop procedure and remove materials
- Ventilate the room, remove the patient to fresh air
- Administer salbutamol
- Call EMS if no improvement

Discussion Questions

- What are common dental office triggers for asthma?
- How can you adapt your operatory to minimize risk?
- How do you decide when to call EMS?

Facilitator Notes

- If the learners forget to remove the patient or ventilate the room, simulate persistent symptoms and rising anxiety.
- If learners hesitate to administer bronchodilators, allow the patient to request their inhaler to prompt action.
- If learners remove the trigger, ventilate, and administer medication early, the patient should respond favorably before EMS arrives.

Pediatric Asthma in the Chair

Overview

A child receiving dental treatment experiences an asthma flare-up during a stressful procedure.

Learning Objectives

- Recognize pediatric asthma signs and symptoms
- Use a metered-dose inhaler with a spacer for children
- Reassure and calm pediatric patients in distress

Setup

Use a pediatric mannequin or a small adult actor. Have a pediatric spacer and a placebo inhaler on hand. Include a caregiver in the room to model realistic interaction.

Clinical Scenario (Narrative)

A 7-year-old boy begins crying and hyperventilating during a cavity filling. The parent says he has "exercise asthma" and uses an inhaler only occasionally.

Patient Presentation

Parameter	Value
Age/Sex	7M
Chief Complaint	Trouble breathing
Onset	During stressful procedure
Vitals	HR: 120, BP: 100/70, RR: 28, SpO_2: 94%
LOC	Awake but panicked
Physical Findings	Suprasternal retractions, wheezing, pale lips

Clinical Course / Timeline

- **0 min**: Child is crying, mild SOB
- **5 min**: Starts gasping, wheezing heard
- **10 min**: Parent gives inhaler, but child can't coordinate the breath
- **15 min**: SpO_2 drops to 89%; lethargy sets in

Critical Actions

- Stop the procedure immediately
- Use a spacer with the inhaler or the clinic-supplied salbutamol
- Provide high-flow oxygen
- Activate EMS and support the airway if needed

Discussion Questions

- What strategies help calm pediatric asthma patients?
- How do you assist with inhaler technique in children?
- When is it appropriate to cancel or postpone treatment?

Facilitator Notes

- If learners fail to involve the parent, have the caregiver become agitated.
- Spacer Technique: Observe whether learners attempt proper pediatric spacer use; offer a cue like, "He usually doesn't take big breaths," if the technique is poor.
- If appropriate emotional and clinical support is provided, the child should calm down and begin improving visibly.

Exercise-Induced Asthma After Climbing Stairs

Overview

A patient becomes short of breath after climbing stairs to your second-floor dental office.

Learning Objectives

- Recognize asthma triggered by exertion
- Support breathing without over-oxygenating
- Know when to escalate based on oxygen saturation

Setup

Have the "patient" enter the clinic visibly winded. Use portable pulse oximeters and an oxygen setup. Simulate stair exertion through brisk walking or jogging in place.

Clinical Scenario (Narrative)

A 61-year-old woman enters the clinic, appearing winded after climbing stairs. She mentions she has asthma but is not concerned. A few minutes later, she begins coughing and holding her chest.

Patient Presentation

Parameter	Value
Age/Sex	61F
Chief Complaint	SOB after exertion
Onset	After climbing stairs
Vitals	HR: 105, BP: 138/88, RR: 24, SpO_2: 91%
LOC	Alert but tired
Physical Findings	Wheezing, pursed-lip breathing, sits hunched forward

Clinical Course / Timeline

- **0 min**: Moderate distress, mild desaturation
- **5 min**: Coughing worsens, difficulty speaking
- **10 min**: SpO_2 drops to 88%, lips slightly blue
- **15 min**: EMS called, patient shaky and exhausted

Critical Actions

- Provide bronchodilator
- Start oxygen
- Sit the patient upright and monitor SpO_2
- Escalate care if no improvement

Discussion Questions

- What makes this different from cardiac exertional symptoms?
- How do you monitor the progression of an asthma attack?
- What level of oxygen support is appropriate in this case?

Facilitator Notes

- If learners hesitate to apply oxygen, simulate a continued drop in SpO_2 and visible signs of fatigue.
- Encourage learners to explain what they're doing to the patient—reward effective communication and reassurance.
- If your training location allows, simulate stairs or exertion to make the scenario more immersive.

Asthma and Anaphylaxis Crossover

Overview

A patient with asthma begins wheezing following the injection of a local anaesthetic, raising concerns of an allergic reaction.

Learning Objectives

- Distinguish between asthma and early anaphylaxis
- Administer epinephrine when appropriate
- Coordinate dual treatment for bronchospasm and allergy

Setup

Use a mannequin or a staff member in a chair. Prepare a mock epinephrine auto-injector, bronchodilator, and oxygen. Simulate facial swelling with moulage or descriptive cues.

Clinical Scenario (Narrative)

A 35-year-old man with asthma is undergoing a root canal. Shortly after receiving lidocaine with epinephrine, he develops tightness in the chest, wheezing, and mild facial flushing.

Patient Presentation

Parameter	Value
Age/Sex	35M
Chief Complaint	Difficulty breathing
Onset	3 minutes after injection
Vitals	HR: 122, BP: 98/60, RR: 26, SpO_2: 93%
LOC	Alert but anxious
Physical Findings	Wheezing, flushed face, scratchy throat

Clinical Course / Timeline

- **0 min**: Mild wheeze, stable vitals
- **5 min**: Throat tightens, BP drops
- **10 min**: Facial swelling starts, SpO_2 drops to 89%
- **15 min**: Patient drowsy, struggling to breathe

Critical Actions

- Recognize a likely allergic reaction
- Administer epinephrine IM (0.3mg adult)
- Provide oxygen and salbutamol
- Activate EMS immediately

Discussion Questions

- When should you give epinephrine vs. salbutamol first?
- What clues help differentiate asthma from anaphylaxis?
- What are your responsibilities while awaiting EMS?

Facilitator Notes

- Withhold full signs of anaphylaxis initially—if learners only treat with salbutamol, progress symptoms toward hypotension and swelling.
- If learners hesitate to give epinephrine, have the patient complain of worsening throat tightness or faintness.
- Use trainer epinephrine devices and simulate real-time decisions about the order of administration.
- If epinephrine is given early with supportive measures, stabilize the patient within 10 minutes and reduce airway symptoms.

Wheezing in the Waiting Room

Overview

A patient with a known history of asthma experiences a sudden exacerbation while waiting for a routine dental cleaning.

Learning Objectives

- Recognize early signs of an asthma exacerbation
- Use a bronchodilator (patient's own or clinic emergency supply) appropriately
- Escalate care when symptoms worsen despite initial treatment

Setup

Use a staff member or a mannequin in a waiting area chair. Place a placebo inhaler (with a spacer) and a simulated oxygen tank with a nasal cannula or mask nearby. Use recorded wheezing sounds if possible.

Clinical Scenario (Narrative)

A 28-year-old woman in the waiting room begins to cough repeatedly and appears short of breath. She tells the receptionist she has asthma and forgot her inhaler.

Patient Presentation

Parameter	Value
Age/Sex	28F
Chief Complaint	Difficulty breathing
Onset	Sudden, while waiting
Vitals	HR: 110, BP: 122/78, RR: 24, SpO_2: 94%
LOC	Alert and anxious
Physical Findings	Audible wheeze, speaks in short phrases, accessory muscle use

Clinical Course / Timeline

- 0 min: Patient is anxious but responsive
- 5 min: Wheezing worsens; speaking is more difficult
- 10 min: SpO_2 drops to 90%; cyanosis begins
- 15 min: EMS not yet arrived; patient slumps in chair

Critical Actions

- Administer salbutamol (via spacer if available)
- Sit the patient upright and provide oxygen
- Activate EMS promptly
- Monitor vitals continuously

Discussion Questions

- When should you administer oxygen vs. a bronchodilator first?
- What are the signs that this patient is progressing to severe asthma?
- What communication steps should you take with EMS?

Facilitator Notes

- Prompting: If learners fail to ask for a bronchodilator early, cue the patient to say, "I forgot my inhaler."
- If no bronchodilator is administered, simulate worsening respiratory distress with increased wheezing, inability to speak in complete sentences, and a drop in SpO_2.
- If learners administer oxygen without also giving a bronchodilator, prompt tachypnea or continued distress to indicate incomplete management.

The Cardiac Arrest Simulations

Cardiac arrest represents the most critical medical emergency a dental team may ever encounter. Although rare, it can occur suddenly and without warning—even in seemingly healthy patients—and requires immediate, coordinated intervention to preserve life. Whether caused by a pre-existing cardiac condition, an adverse drug reaction, severe hypoxia, or another medical event, cardiac arrest demands that all members of the dental team respond with confidence, speed, and precision.

Survival from cardiac arrest depends heavily on the early recognition of unresponsiveness, rapid activation of emergency medical services, initiation of high-quality cardiopulmonary resuscitation (CPR), and timely use of an automated external defibrillator (AED). In the dental setting, delays in identifying arrest or initiating adequate resuscitation can result in irreversible outcomes.

Dental professionals are not expected to function as emergency physicians, but they are ethically and professionally responsible for initiating life-saving interventions until EMS arrives. Simulating cardiac arrest scenarios ensures that providers are mentally, emotionally, and technically prepared to act when seconds matter most.

Why Include Cardiac Arrest in Simulation Training?

Cardiac arrest is the highest-stakes, lowest-frequency event in dental practice. It tests the readiness of the entire team, not just their clinical skills, but their ability to function effectively under extreme pressure. Simulation offers a controlled environment to prepare for this rare but devastating emergency.

A cardiac arrest simulation:

- Develops fluency in basic life support (BLS). Simulation reinforces high-quality chest compressions, effective rescue breathing, and proper rotation of team members to avoid fatigue. It helps translate BLS theory into rapid, real-world action.

- Ensures familiarity with emergency equipment. Teams gain hands-on experience locating and using emergency tools such as the AED, oxygen system, bag-valve-mask (BVM), and emergency medications. Practice builds muscle memory and reduces hesitancy during real crises.

- Improves role clarity and team dynamics. Cardiac arrest simulations clarify who performs compressions, who manages the airway, who retrieves the AED, and who calls 911. This fosters efficient role delegation and minimizes confusion under pressure.

- Builds confidence in high-stress situations.

Emotional stress is high during real resuscitation efforts. Simulation enables teams to experience stress in a safe setting, developing composure, confidence, and effective communication strategies.

Although we hope never to encounter cardiac arrest in a dental office, preparation is essential. These simulations are designed to help your team recognize cardiac arrest early, act decisively, and deliver high-quality resuscitation in those critical first minutes—actions that can mean the difference between life and death.

Post-Operative Syncope Turns to Arrest

Overview

A middle-aged woman faints while standing post-procedure. She initially recovers, then arrests moments later. Learners must recognize a deteriorating patient and respond.

Learning Objectives

- Recognize vasovagal syncope and red flags for deterioration
- Ensure safety after fainting episodes
- Respond to sudden cardiac arrest in an upright patient

Setup

Use a standing CPR mannequin or have an actor "collapse" from standing. Use a reclining chair for recovery, then simulate a second collapse.

Clinical Scenario (Narrative)

A 52-year-old woman faints after standing up post-filling. She is laid back and recovers. While preparing to discharge, she seizes briefly and arrests.

Patient Presentation

Parameter	Value
Age/Sex	52F
Chief Complaint	Lightheadedness
Onset	After standing
Vitals	Initially normal, then unresponsive
LOC	Brief LOC, then alert, then unresponsive
Physical Findings	Pale, diaphoretic, seizure-like activity

Clinical Course / Timeline

- **0 min**: Collapse from standing, regains consciousness
- **3 min**: Still pale, feeling "weird"
- **5 min**: Becomes unresponsive, no pulse
- **6 min**: CPR initiated

Critical Actions

- Monitor closely after syncope
- Use positioning to prevent further collapse
- Recognize seizure as a possible pre-arrest sign
- Initiate BLS immediately

Discussion Questions

- What distinguishes benign fainting from a more dangerous loss of consciousness?
- How should a post-faint patient be monitored?
- How can a dental chair be used to protect patients from injury?

Facilitator Notes

- Cue for early signs of deterioration if learners are observant
- Introduce confusion with seizure activity if needed

Anaphylaxis to Local Anaesthetic Leading to Arrest

Overview

A young adult develops anaphylaxis moments after receiving local anaesthetic. The team must recognize and treat the reaction and manage a resulting cardiac arrest.

Learning Objectives

- Identify signs of anaphylaxis
- Administer intramuscular epinephrine
- Manage airway swelling and respiratory distress
- Transition to cardiac arrest management

Setup

Use a mannequin in the dental chair. Prepare mock epinephrine auto-injectors or IM syringes. Simulate stridor and wheezing through audio.

Clinical Scenario (Narrative)

A 28-year-old female receives 2% lidocaine with epinephrine. Within one minute, she complains of throat tightness, difficulty breathing, and itchy skin. Rapid deterioration follows.

Patient Presentation

Parameter	Value
Age/Sex	28F
Chief Complaint	Swelling, shortness of breath
Onset	1–2 minutes post-injection
Vitals	HR: 110, BP: 88/50, RR: 26, SpO$_2$: 92%
LOC	Anxious, semi-alert, then unresponsive
Physical Findings	Wheezing, facial swelling, rash

Clinical Course / Timeline

- **0 min**: Patient complains of swelling, itchy throat
- **1 min**: Stridor, wheezing, hypotension
- **2 min**: IM epinephrine given
- **3 min**: LOC deteriorates, cardiac arrest ensues
- **4 min**: CPR started, AED attached

Critical Actions

- Recognize anaphylaxis and give IM epinephrine
- Call 911 early
- Maintain airway, provide oxygen
- Transition to BLS when the patient arrests
- Record the timing of epinephrine and events

Discussion Questions

- What are the early vs. late signs of anaphylaxis?
- What is the correct dose and route for epinephrine?
- What medications must be immediately accessible in every dental office?

Facilitator Notes

- Allow different team members to "notice" the rash, wheeze, or hypotension
- Vary the timing of arrest based on learner actions

Sudden Collapse in the Waiting Room

Overview

A patient in the waiting room collapses. The team must transition from administrative mode to emergency response, activating emergency protocols and performing BLS.

Learning Objectives

- Transition rapidly from clinical to emergency roles
- Identify cardiac arrest in a non-clinical space
- Communicate clearly under pressure
- Manage bystander involvement and initiate BLS

Setup

Place a mannequin in a waiting room chair. One actor collapses to the floor. Assign staff to simulate reception and dental team roles.

Clinical Scenario (Narrative)

A 45-year-old male in the waiting room, waiting for a hygiene appointment, slumps in his chair and slides to the ground. A receptionist witnesses this and calls for help.

Patient Presentation

Parameter	Value
Age/Sex	45M
Chief Complaint	None prior to collapse
Onset	Sudden, unwitnessed
Vitals	No pulse, not breathing
LOC	Unresponsive
Physical Findings	No movement, pale, cool skin

Clinical Course / Timeline

- **0 min**: Unresponsive and pulseless
- **1 min**: CPR started, AED fetched
- **3 min**: AED arrives and first shock advised
- **5 min**: Continued CPR, second shock
- **8 min**: EMS arrival

Critical Actions

- Recognize unresponsiveness and assess pulse
- Activate EMS
- Retrieve and apply an AED
- Perform continuous BLS
- Communicate clearly and document the event

Discussion Questions

- How would you ensure rapid AED access in all clinic areas?
- How should front desk staff be trained for emergencies?
- How do you manage bystanders or other patients during a crisis?

Facilitator Notes

- Add background noise (phones, waiting patients) for realism
- Include a mock "child" in the waiting area to test distraction management

Collapse During Nitrous Oxide Sedation

Overview

A patient under nitrous oxide for anxiety suddenly becomes apneic and pulseless. Learners must recognize overdose or apnea, discontinue nitrous oxide, and begin CPR.

Learning Objectives

- Recognize respiratory depression during sedation
- Discontinue nitrous oxide and administer 100% oxygen
- Initiate CPR and AED use when needed
- Understand sedation monitoring limitations in dental offices

Setup

Simulate a nitrous oxide delivery system with dials or empty tanks. Use a CPR mannequin with an oxygen mask and a nasal hood.

Clinical Scenario (Narrative)

A 33-year-old male receiving nitrous oxide for a crown prep becomes still and pale. He stops responding and has no palpable pulse.

Patient Presentation

Parameter	Value
Age/Sex	33M
Chief Complaint	Anxiety, undergoing sedation
Onset	10 minutes into sedation
Vitals	Apneic, pulseless
LOC	Unresponsive
Physical Findings	No chest rise, cyanosis

Clinical Course / Timeline

- **0 min**: Observed apnea
- **1 min**: Attempted stimulation fails
- **2 min**: Pulseless, AED attached
- **3 min**: CPR and first shock delivered

Critical Actions

- Stop nitrous oxide and give 100% oxygen
- Assess responsiveness and pulse
- Initiate CPR and call EMS
- Monitor oxygen delivery and airway

Discussion Questions

- How do you recognize sedation-related emergencies?
- What is the role of oxygen during and after nitrous oxide use?
- How should sedated patients be monitored?

Facilitator Notes

- Vary nitrous oxide flow rates in the scenario to test awareness
- Reinforce the need for suction, airway management readiness

Cardiac Arrest During Tooth Extraction

Overview

A healthy-appearing adult male collapses suddenly during a routine dental extraction. The team must recognize cardiac arrest, begin high-quality CPR, and use an AED without delay.

Learning Objectives

- Recognize sudden cardiac arrest in the dental chair
- Initiate high-quality chest compressions and ventilation
- Operate an AED appropriately in a clinical environment
- Coordinate roles and maintain effective team communication

Setup

Use a CPR mannequin in a dental chair. One person acts as the dentist, and others as dental staff. Use a real or trainer AED. Simulate suction and oxygen use with props or available equipment.

Clinical Scenario (Narrative)

During a simple tooth extraction on a 62-year-old male, the patient gasped and became unresponsive. There is no pulse. A dental assistant calls out, "Doctor, he's not breathing!"

Patient Presentation

Parameter	Value
Age/Sex	62M
Chief Complaint	Routine extraction
Onset	Sudden collapse during procedure
Vitals	Pulseless, apneic
LOC	Unresponsive (GCS 3)
Physical Findings	Cyanotic lips, limp body

Clinical Course / Timeline

- **0 min**: Collapse, pulseless
- **1 min**: AED attached, advises shock
- **2 min**: Shock delivered, CPR resumed
- **4 min**: EMS called, airway supported with BVM
- **6 min**: ROSC or no change, depending on actions

Critical Actions

- Call for help / activate EMS
- Begin CPR within 10 seconds
- Attach and use an AED as soon as available
- Provide effective BVM ventilation with oxygen
- Rotate compressors every 2 minutes

Discussion Questions

- What are the immediate signs of cardiac arrest?
- How should tasks be delegated in a dental emergency?
- What are common errors during BLS that reduce effectiveness?
- How often should a dental office rehearse code drills?

Facilitator Notes (Optional)

- Delay AED availability to test prioritization
- Introduce a family member on scene if learners stall
- Reinforce CPR quality and team dynamics

Preparing the Dental Office for Emergencies

Let's face it—medical emergencies are rare in the dental office, but when they do happen, they can be intense and fast-moving. The difference between a smooth response and a chaotic one often comes down to preparation. Think of it like fire drills in school: you hope you'll never need them, but if you do, you'll be glad you practiced.

So, how do you prepare your dental office for those unexpected moments? It starts with a bit of planning and a lot of teamwork.

First, take a step back and consider the kinds of emergencies your team is most likely to see. Syncope (fainting), allergic reactions, chest pain, and even cardiac events can all occur, especially in a busy practice with a diverse patient population. Knowing what you might face helps you focus your training and resources where they'll have the most impact.

Next, it's essential to have clear, written protocols. These aren't just for show; they're your playbook for when things go sideways. Who calls 911? Who grabs the emergency kit? Who manages the patient's airway? When everyone knows their role, you avoid the confusion that can cost precious seconds. Ensure that these protocols are easily accessible and that new staff members receive training on them right away.

However, having a plan isn't enough; you must practice it. That's where regular drills come in. Just like you wouldn't expect a hockey team to win without practicing, you can't expect your team to handle emergencies smoothly without rehearsing. Monthly simulations, even just 15 minutes long, help everyone stay sharp and confident. And don't forget to mix things up—sometimes change the scenario or the roles — so everyone gets comfortable with different responsibilities.

Communication is another big piece of the puzzle. In an emergency, clear and calm communication can make all the difference. Ensure your team knows how to communicate effectively with each other and with emergency responders. Post important phone numbers and your office address in a visible location, and practice giving a quick and accurate report to EMS.

Your office environment matters, too. Emergency equipment should be easy to find and clearly labelled. Make it a habit to check your supplies regularly—nothing's worse than reaching for a piece of equipment and finding it missing or expired. Keep pathways clear for quick access and ensure everyone knows where the emergency exits are located.

Finally, keep the momentum going. Emergency preparedness isn't a one-and-done deal. Keep records of your drills, note what worked and what didn't, and update your protocols as you learn. Celebrate successes and learn from mistakes, but above all, make sure everyone feels empowered to speak up and ask questions.

When you weave all these elements together—planning,

practice, communication, and continuous improvement—
you create a team that's not just ready for emergencies,
but confident and calm under pressure. That's something
your patients will notice and appreciate.

Preparing a Medical Emergency Kit for the Dental Office

A well-prepared medical emergency kit is the cornerstone of effective emergency response in the dental office. This chapter outlines practical steps for assembling, maintaining, and utilizing a kit tailored to your practice's needs, ensuring readiness for the most common emergencies.

Every office will have different needs and capabilities, so no two kits will be the same, but here are some common components of a Dental Office Emergency Kit that you should consider including in yours:

Basic Life Support Equipment
- Automated External Defibrillator (AED)
- Bag-valve-mask (BVM) device
- Oxygen tank and delivery systems (nasal cannulas, masks)
- Suction device and tubing
- Blood pressure cuff and stethoscope
- Medical gloves

Emergency Medications
- Epinephrine auto-injector or ampoule
- Nitroglycerine (tablets or spray)
- Oral glucose gel or tablets

- Aspirin (for suspected cardiac events)
- Antihistamine (e.g. diphenhydramine)

Airway Management Supplies
- Oropharyngeal airways (various sizes)
- Nasopharyngeal airways
- Pocket mask with one-way valve
- Monitoring and Diagnostic Tools
- Pulse oximeter

Miscellaneous Supplies
- Gloves, gauze, and adhesive tape
- Syringes and needles (for medication administration if trained)
- Emergency contact numbers and protocols
- Glucometer and test strips

Kit Organization and Maintenance

An effective emergency kit is essential; however, merely possessing one is not sufficient. If the kit is stored away in a closet or lacks necessary items, it will be of little use when a crisis arises. Therefore, maintaining your emergency kit in an organized and current state is crucial.

Start by choosing a central spot for your emergency kit— somewhere everyone on the team can find it quickly, even in a rush. Consider the flow of your office and select a location that's easily accessible, such as a cabinet in the main operatory or a dedicated shelf in the staff room. Make sure it's clearly labelled so there's no confusion about what's inside.

Now, who's in charge of keeping things in order? Consider assigning a staff member the role of "Emergency Supplies Coordinator". This person checks the kit each month, ensuring that nothing has expired or is missing, and maintains a simple log of what has been checked and when. It doesn't have to be a big job, but having one person responsible means the kit doesn't get forgotten.

Training is just as important as the kit itself. Everyone on the team should know where the kit is, what's inside, and how to use the key items. Make it part of your regular emergency drills by practicing how to grab the kit, check the supplies, and use the equipment. That way, if an emergency happens, everyone knows exactly what to do.

Safety and Compliance

Here's a rule to live by: never mix training supplies with the real deal. It's far too easy to accidentally grab a training-only item in the heat of the moment, so ensure everything in your emergency kit is clearly marked for real emergencies. For your training props, attach a large "TRAINING ONLY" label on them and store them in a completely different spot.

Infection control is important, even during training. If you are using mannequins or airway devices that multiple people handle, ensure they are cleaned after each use. Store your moulage makeup and other reusable props in sealed containers to maintain hygiene and ensure they are ready for the next drill.

By keeping your kit organized, well-maintained, and safe, you're not just checking a box—you're ensuring your team is truly prepared to handle whatever comes their way. That peace of mind is worth its weight in gold.

By following these guidelines, your dental office will have a reliable, ready-to-use emergency kit that supports rapid, effective response to medical crises, reinforcing your commitment to patient safety and care.

Conclusion
A General Approach to Emergencies

When it comes to managing emergencies in the dental office, there's no single magic formula. What really makes a difference is cultivating a culture in which preparation, teamwork, and adaptability are integral to everyday practice. While it's tempting to focus on the latest equipment or the most advanced protocols, the real strength lies in how well your team collaborates under pressure.

Consider this: emergencies, by their very nature, are unpredictable. You may have a patient who suddenly feels dizzy, another who has an allergic reaction, or, in rare instances, someone whose heart stops. In those moments, it's not just about who knows what to do—it's about how the entire team responds, communicates, and supports one another. That's why regular training and open communication are so crucial. They help everyone remain calm, focused, and prepared to act.

Preparation is the foundation. By practicing emergency scenarios together, your team becomes familiar with their roles, the location of critical supplies, and the steps to take when things go awry. This kind of routine builds confidence, ensuring that when a real emergency occurs, muscle memory takes over, and panic doesn't have a chance to set in. It's not unlike learning a new skill—repetition and reflection are key. After each drill, taking a few minutes to debrief and discuss what went well and what could be improved helps everyone learn and grow.

Teamwork and communication are the glue that holds everything together. In the heat of the moment, clear, concise communication can mean the difference between confusion and coordinated action. Encouraging everyone to speak up, ask questions, and share ideas creates an environment where people feel empowered to help, not just follow orders. And when the team works well together, patients and their families feel reassured, even in stressful situations.

Adaptability is just as important as preparation. No two emergencies are exactly alike, and sometimes things don't go as planned. Being able to think on your feet, adjust your approach, and learn from each experience sets truly prepared teams apart. That's why it's so valuable to review and update your protocols regularly, incorporating new knowledge and insights from both simulations and real-life events.

Ultimately, the goal is to provide the best possible care for your patients, even in the most challenging circumstances. By integrating emergency preparedness into your office culture, you create a practice that is not only safer but also more resilient and confident. Patients notice when a team is calm, competent, and caring—and that trust is something money cannot buy.

As you move forward, remember that emergencies are rare, but readiness is always essential. Continue practicing, continue communicating, and continue learning. That's the best way to ensure your dental office is prepared for anything that comes your way.

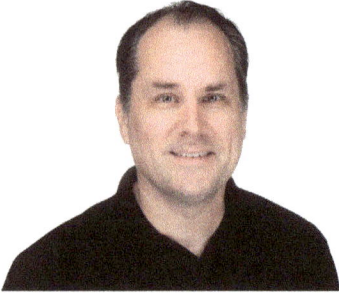

About the Author

Trystan brings a wealth of real-world emergency medicine experience to his writing, shaped by a career spent at the sharp end of critical care, rescue, and medical education. With decades of frontline service as an advanced paramedic and flight paramedic, Trystan has not only responded to countless emergencies but has also trained generations of healthcare professionals—including doctors, paramedics, dentists, nurses, and Canadian Air Force Search and Rescue technicians.

His leadership has extended far beyond the ambulance and helicopter: Trystan managed a large, remote clinic staffed by nurse practitioners, physician assistants, registered nurses, paramedics, laboratory technicians, and X-ray technologists. Throughout several tumultuous years of the COVID-19 pandemic, he led this enormous and complex operation as both manager and senior clinician, orchestrating care amid unprecedented challenges and ensuring his team was prepared for anything, from routine health needs to life-threatening emergencies.

Trystan's background is uniquely broad. He has served as

a fire chief for several years, blending emergency management with community leadership. His passion for adventure and safety has led him to roles as a ski patroller, lifeguard, and even a professional scuba diver (funny story!). Currently, Trystan is spearheading a project to bring hyperbaric emergency medicine to remote regions, working in partnership with the helicopter EMS (HEMS) operation, where he continues to provide advanced medical care and technical rescue.

Academically, Trystan holds a degree in biology and is soon to complete a master's degree in medical education —a testament to his commitment to both the science and the teaching of emergency care. Throughout his career, Trystan has remained dedicated to sharing knowledge, improving systems, and empowering teams to respond with confidence and skill.

Trystan's book on preparing dental offices for emergencies draws on his extensive experience in simulation-based training, interprofessional teamwork, and emergency response. He believes that the best outcomes come from preparation, clear communication, and a culture of continuous learning—principles that have guided his work across emergency medical services, firefighting, and remote healthcare.

References

1. Reid J, Stone K, Brown J, et al. The Simulation Team Assessment Tool (STAT): development, reliability and validation. Resuscitation. 2012;83(7):879-886. doi:10.1016/j.resuscitation.2011.12.012

2. Kolb DA. Experiential learning: experience as the source of learning and development. Englewood Cliffs, NJ: Prentice-Hall; 1984.

3. Okuyama Y, Sugiura Y, Ikegami A, et al. Incidence and characteristics of medical emergencies related to dental treatment: a single-center retrospective study. J Oral Sci. 2021;63(2):160-166. doi:10.2334/josnusd.20-0417

4. Schöpper M, Götzinger A, Steinhausen N, et al. Dental care in patients with epilepsy: a survey of 82 patients and their dentists. J Oral Sci. 2020;62(4):511-518. doi:10.2334/josnusd.20-0417

5. Smereka J, Aluchna M, Aluchna A, et al. Medical emergencies in dental hygienists' practice. Medicine (Baltimore). 2019;98(30):e16613.

6. Cooke M. Cerebrovascular accident under anesthesia during dental alveolar surgery: case report and anesthesia management. Anesth Prog. 2013;60(4):164-170. doi:10.2344/0003-3006-60.4.164

7. Baghani E, Ouanounou A. The dental management of the asthmatic patients. Spec Care Dentist. 2021;41(3):309-318. doi:10.1111/scd.12566

www.ingramcontent.com/pod-product-compliance
Lightning Source LLC
Chambersburg PA
CBHW051257020426
42333CB00026B/3238